INSTANT
INTUITION

INSTANT INTUITION

A psychic's guide to finding answers
to life's important questions

Foreword by Paul McKenna

ANNE JIRSCH

piatkus

PIATKUS

First published in Great Britain in 2007 by Piatkus
This paperback edition published in 2008 by Piatkus
Reprinted 2009, 2010

A CIP catalogue record for this book
is available from the British Library.

ISBN 978-0-7499-2921-3

Typeset in Perpetua by Action Publishing Technology Ltd, Gloucester
Printed and bound in Great Britain by
Clays Ltd, St Ives plc

Papers used by Piatkus are natural, renewable and
recyclable products sourced from well-managed forests and certified
in accordance with the rules of the Forest Stewardship Council.

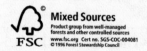

Mixed Sources
Product group from well-managed
forests and other controlled sources
www.fsc.org Cert no. SGS-COC-004081
© 1996 Forest Stewardship Council

Piatkus
An imprint of
Little, Brown Book Group
100 Victoria Embankment
London EC4Y 0DY

An Hachette UK Company
www.hachette.co.uk

www.piatkus.co.uk

Contents

Acknowledgements

I would like to thank:

Paul McKenna, an inspiration and the kindest and cleverest person I know.

Paul Duddridge for his advice and occasional kick in the right place.

Clare Staples for her support and back up.

Robert Kirby and Judy Piatkus for believing in me.

And Monica Cafferky for burning the midnight oil and for her dedication to the project.

Also, the following people need a special thank you for permissions granted to quote from their work or for giving their time for interviews: Skip Atwater; Cleve Backster, author of *Primary Perception: Biocommunication with Plants, Living Foods and Human Cells* (White Rose Millennium Press, 2003); Bruce E. Calkins from Moller International; Carmen Clews and Charlie Wright; Tammy Delph; Kelly and Stacey Franklin; Malcolm Gladwell, author of *Blink: The Power of Thinking Without Thinking* (Allen Lane, Penguin Group, 2005); Dr Harry Oldfield, author of *Invisible Universe* (Thorsons, 1998); Chris Robinson and Dr Keith Hearne; Dr Dean Radin, author of *The Conscious Universe* (HarperCollins, 1997); Greg Secker; and Colin Wilson.

Foreword

In the mid-1990s, I made a television series about the 'paranormal' – those things that exist outside of the realm of what most of us have experienced in our own lives. Until that time, I had been very sceptical about the whole idea of 'psychic phenomena', but over the months of filming I saw so many unusual and inexplicable things for myself that I had to open up to the possibility that there was more to it than I had previously thought. In fact, several of the psychics I met during the filming of the show were so accurate and seemed to have such intimate knowledge of my past (and future!) that my beliefs about what is possible for the well-trained mind changed for ever.

A number of years later, a psychologist friend of mine called and said, 'I saw an amazing psychic recently – you're into all that weirdy stuff, aren't you?' This surprised me, since my friend came from a scientific background and was usually sceptical of anything that didn't fit into the rigid categories of psychology or science. Indeed, she admitted to me that she had initially gone along to see if she could catch the psychic out by making up false people and situations and asking about them as if they were real. Each time she asked a fake question, the psychic told her that the people and situations didn't exist and went on to give her real and intimate insights into the various areas of her life – relationships, finances and career – with extraordinary accuracy.

That psychic was Anne Jirsch, and within an hour of meeting her I was a fan. What really impressed me was not just her intuitive and predictive ability as a psychic, but that, given her background as a therapist, she was able to offer advice that didn't just answer my questions, but moved me to a more empowered place from which to deal with the challenges in my life.

Over the years, Anne has consistently offered me extremely helpful advice about business, relationships and myself. If anyone ever rolls their eyes and tells me that they think it's 'unusual' that I consult a psychic, I simply say that I employ accountants, lawyers and agents to give me advice – why not a psychic if she is truly skilled at her craft? Indeed, a great number of high-achievers and celebrities in the world of business and the arts regularly consult with her as well.

More than anything I can say about her abilities as a psychic and therapist, Anne is a genuinely good person – and that shines through in every page of this wonderful book.

It is my sincere hope that reading this book and doing Anne's exercises will give you insight into your own psychic potential and open your mind to the limitless possibilities that are within you!

Paul McKenna

INSTANT INTUITION

CHAPTER 1

Switching On Your Psychic Antennae

In the backstreets of Notting Hill, London, where I grew up, no one was ambitious. Most of my classmates were destined to work in a factory, although the few clever ones might land an office job. My best friend wanted to work in a shoe shop and my cousin dreamed of being a hairdresser. Me? I just wanted to be psychic. I wanted to be like my gran, who I spent wonderful summer holidays with in Kent. Every August, Mum and I would travel by train from London to Orpington, where Gran lived. For six weeks I entered her world of magic, mystery and fortune telling.

Winny was originally from the East End and always had time to pop the kettle on and listen to people's problems and look into their futures. I remember an endless stream of women knocking on her front door and asking, 'Winny, would you read the tea leaves for me?' or 'Win, will you buy my wart?' She would then give them a penny for their wart. The next day their unsightly lump would have vanished but Gran would have a tiny brown mark on her finger which would disappear within 48 hours.

Staying with Gran was exciting because each day was so different. Sometimes she would wake me up just before dawn and say, 'Quick, let's go and pick mushrooms.' She told me that the mushrooms played games with us. They would pop out of the ground behind us teasingly. She was right. We would carefully look at a piece of grass to check it was fungi-free. Then, as we walked away, we would glance back and find several mushrooms.

While I picked mushrooms on the school playing fields at the back of her council house, my grandmother would gather wild herbs. But I never knew what she did with these ingredients. My herbal training was very basic. I was only allowed to pick mint to put in with the new potatoes.

My deaf grandfather also had a gift, or so we first thought, when he began to hear voices. He told me, 'I can hear all this talking but I can't make out a word. It's so annoying.' Even at my young age – I was nine at the time – I thought it was odd that my granddad's poor hearing could affect his ability to hear spirit messages.

One day, Granddad was snoozing in his favourite armchair when we heard loud music. 'Where's that coming from?' asked my Uncle Joe. It was coming from Granddad, and we were both baffled. We could distinctly hear Elvis. Later, we discovered his hearing aid was picking up the local radio station. I think he told me stories about the 'spirit voices' because he just wanted to be psychic like Gran. I know I certainly wanted her skills because she helped people, and her 'clients' always left the house happier. 'What a great job!' I thought.

Over the years I watched my grandmother read the tea leaves for hundreds of people. She always spoke with great authority and was a walking encyclopaedia of solutions to people's problems. She also knew everything that went on in Orpington. I overheard gossip about affairs, backstreet abortions and who owed the pawnbroker a fortune. Life was not easy in those days, but it was colourful.

These days, Winny would be called a 'role model', but to me she was my wonderful gran – someone I looked up to and admired. I would sit on the end of my bed and concentrate and try to have a premonition. I would think, 'Right, there's going to be a train crash' or 'I can see an earthquake in China.' Even with the laws of chance, I should have made at least one correct prediction. But at that point in my life I wasn't tuned into my clairvoyant powers, my Instant Intuition. This awakening came later.

My mother was a shining example of someone who used her natural psychic talents, but unlike Gran, she never developed them to their full potential. Mum viewed her gift as a bit of fun rather than a way of making a living. Her job was running a local petrol station. All the locals used the garage and anyone who was pregnant would be instructed by a family member, 'Go and see Sylvie – she'll tell you whether it's a boy or girl.' My mother would take the woman's wedding ring and thread it onto her own gold chain, which she wore around her neck. She would then hold this makeshift pendulum over the lady's hand and wait for it to move. If the wedding ring and chain circled in a clockwise direction the child would be a girl, and if it moved anti-clockwise the woman was expecting a boy.

My mum was always right. On the strength of her prediction the pregnant woman would then go and buy pink or blue baby clothes and announce to everyone the sex of her unborn child. My mother also had healing hands, but when Gran ever mentioned it she flatly denied any knowledge of this gift. However, when her precious Jack Russell, Susie, was dying,

Mum laid her hands on her for hours. The next day the twelve year old dog suddenly stood up, walked around the room, then jumped onto her lap. Susie lived another five years.

Throughout my teens, with Gran's and Mum's skills taunting me, I continued with my attempts to be psychic, but nothing ever happened. Now I realise this was because I was trying too hard and I had no idea how to tune into my Instant Intuition. I was gifted, it ran in my blood, but my psychic antennae weren't switched on. It was as if I was watching a film with the sound turned off and only picking up half of the story. During the 20 years I've been teaching and running psychic-development workshops, I've met many people who have had the same experience. It's actually very common for novices to struggle with their spiritual gifts at first because they don't know how to tune in. But once you switch on using the simple techniques outlined in this book, this initial barrier will be an easy one to overcome.

As well as developing an interest in clairvoyance, I had a thirst for travel, which was unusual for my area. I lived in Notting Hill before it became fashionable and upmarket. To be frank, it was a slum. There were no organic delis and boutiques then. Instead, women walked around with their hair in curlers covered by headscarves. Everything was on tick, meaning you bought your groceries, clothes and furniture and paid for the goods when you had the cash. And everyone owed cash to the moneylender, or 'tallyman', as we called him.

It was a rough area, so it was a cheap place to live. When the West Indians were invited over by the Government in the 1950s to work on the buses and in the factories and hospitals, many of them flocked to Notting Hill. From what I remember, the integration of the white and black communities was relatively smooth. We were fascinated with the food they ate and their bright, colourful clothes.

Having people from such a faraway country on hand to chat to was fascinating for me. As a street urchin hanging around outside my house, I was in a prime position to strike up conversations with my West Indian neighbours, who were happy to talk about their homeland. I heard about the heat, the food, the wildlife, the beaches, and it seemed so different from damp and dark Britain. I had to explore this other world, the world outside London, and this urge burned inside me.

At that time it was rare for people to venture any further than Spain, but I wanted to see the world. When I hit my teens I fantasised about going to India, China and beyond. I had a friend called Charlie who disappeared to India for two years. He returned to Slough, where I was now living, full of amazing stories. Charlie told me about the temples and the strange spicy food. I sat transfixed in our local pub as he recounted encounters with mystics and told tales of meeting rebels high in the hills in Afghanistan. Later, Charlie admitted that he exaggerated his stories. Even so, by then he had fired my imagination. I had caught the wanderlust bug.

So at the tender age of eighteen, I packed my rucksack and headed East with £100 in my pocket. Nowadays it's normal to travel abroad, and every high street is thriving with restaurants selling world cuisine. But 30 years ago I had never eaten a curry, and Slough only had a handful of Italian restaurants and an abundance of greasy-spoon cafés. I was heading into the unknown, gastronomically and spiritually.

My mum was not amused that I wanted to travel – gap years were not the norm in 1972. Newspapers were full of stories of 'dropouts' in India taking drugs. Only four years before, in

1968, the Beatles had visited the country and put it firmly on the hippie trail. When my Aunt Mabel heard about my plans, she told Mum, 'The English kids in India are lying in the gutters. They're smoking mari-jew-ana. You can't let her go.' But I was eighteen and legally free to do what I wanted, so I talked to the experienced travellers and planned my trip. Later I caught the train from London to Istanbul and Gran's parting words echoed in my ears, 'Good for you, girl. If I was younger I'd join you.'

My psychic adventure

Once in Istanbul, I booked into my hotel then headed to the Pudding Shop, which is still open today. It sells puddings and strong black tea known as chai, and it was like a tourist information centre with people hitching rides in beaten-up Volkswagen vans from Turkey to Asia. The famous Magic Bus operated from the shop, and this is how I travelled for two weeks from Istanbul to Kabul in Afghanistan.

Afghanistan has a strange energy. It's like no other place I had ever visited. No matter how organised, everyone forgets their routine in this country. It's as if time stopped. I found myself really thinking about life and why we were here on this earth. As a child I was curious about religion and spirituality, and now, in this exotic far-off land, as I sat in chai houses sipping my black tea I began to ask myself the big questions. Why are we here? Is our life preordained or do we create our own reality? Have I lived before?

By the time I reached India I was ready for some answers and ready to open my psychic mind. Within days, fate answered my wish and I met a Hindu holy man at a temple, who told me about the god Krishna fighting a seven-headed serpent. It sounded daft. I asked him, 'Surely you don't really believe all that nonsense?' He quickly replied, 'Do you believe after death there's nothing else?' It suddenly struck me that maybe everything I had been brought up to believe was nonsense. I began the quest to find myself and the truth.

I stayed at ashrams, meditated with Buddhists and prayed at temples. I visited the Bodhi Tree, in northern India, where Buddha sat and gained his enlightenment. But on this trip my greatest spiritual teacher was a beggar I met in Calcutta. I know I should be telling you about a great guru wearing pure white flowing robes, but the beggar had all the answers to my big questions. More importantly, he taught me how to switch on my psychic gifts and my Instant Intuition.

I had been in Calcutta for five days when I struck up a conversation with the beggar in the street. He was sitting on his dusty straw mat leaning against a kiosk that sold drinks and cigarettes. He had long grey hair, a straggly beard and ragged dirty clothes that must have once been white. His dirty feet were bare. Every morning I had passed him on my way to buy my breakfast of tea and chapati from a café. On the fifth day I said hello and we began chatting. He told me his name was Vikram.

Vikram had an easy manner and it was clear everyone liked him. As I squatted in the dusty street, the locals all greeted him as they walked past. Observing how others spoke to him, I soon realised that although this man was a beggar, he commanded respect. I began taking him his breakfast and as he ate we talked about spirituality. Vikram was full of tales about the afterlife, reincarnation and karma. He liked telling stories. This was his way of passing on information and encouraging debate.

All day Vikram sat on his mat and people flocked to him. He had charisma. He never worried where his next meal was coming from and he taught me how to gain inner peace. Any other person would have been driven mad by my constant questions, but Vikram loved a challenge. Every afternoon for the remaining five weeks I stayed in Calcutta I went to see him. I would squat down on the dust, shaded by the canopy of the kiosk, and we'd chat. I would ask him questions like, 'So, why don't you have a job?' Vikram would reply, 'What for? I am provided with everything I need by the people who come to see me.'

My Western mind programming would then take over: 'But don't you want to better yourself?' Vikram would laugh and ask me, 'What is bettering oneself? How do you define that?' A good question.

'I don't know, buy a house,' I would say with a shrug.

'I don't need a house. I live here in the street. If I lived in a house I would never see all of these wonderful people, my friends.'

He swept his hand out in front of his body in a big arc. The people passing turned and smiled at him. Every day they left him food and money on his mat and he would exchange a few words with them. He lifted their spirits and often gave them advice about their problems. Each morning I continued to take him tea and chapattis, which was my way of thanking him for his company.

Our conversations were peppered by the beeps of motorbike horns and the noise of the streets of Calcutta. With the colourful mayhem all around us Vikram taught me that the only peace you can ever experience is the stillness within yourself. Other people cannot make you happy, nor can money or possessions. He told me, 'If you shut up long enough, if you still your monkey mind, you can ask and receive answers to any question.' He instructed me how to relax in order to quieten that 'monkey mind' (so-called because, like a monkey in the jungle jumping from tree to tree, the mind jumps restlessly from thought to thought, never settling, never focusing). Once my monkey mind was settled, I was supposed to use the pictures in my mind to find the answers to my questions.

I doubt that I was quiet for more than 30 seconds during the whole time I spent with him. As for the mind pictures, I had no idea what he was talking about. He was a very patient man. But later his words flooded back to me and the seeds he had planted flourished. As I switched on my own Instant Intuition, I developed an invaluable technique that I call 'The Album', which is based on Vikram's teachings. It's a simple and effective exercise, which you will find later in this chapter.

Despite my wonderful experiences with Vikram, backpacking took some getting used to because it was such an alien way to live after being accustomed to a bed and four walls. It was also odd being cut off from the news and 'real life', but we still had books and swapped battered volumes with people we bumped into along the way. I met an American in a coffee shop who gladly gave me a 'novel full of mystical shit'. The book was *The Teachings of Don Juan* by Carlos Castaneda. I wish I could tell you that I picked up on the parallels between Castaneda's book and what was happening in my life right then, but in truth it went straight over my head. In fact, it was probably over 20 years later that it dawned on me that while I was reading about Carlos's trip to Mexico – where he met an Indian shaman to whom he became an apprentice and learned secret knowledge – I'd had a similar experience myself with Vikram.

As I sat on the beach in Goa watching the most beautiful sunset I had ever seen, I read about Don Juan's teachings. As

Vikram taught me about 'seeing', Carlos spoke about Don Juan's exasperation as he tried to teach him the difference between 'looking' and 'seeing'. Even though I missed the synchronicity, the book fascinated me and it opened up a whole new way of thinking about life and energy. And although Vikram and Don Juan used very different words to teach, the message was very similar. I read Don Juan's words, 'The twilight is the crack between the worlds.' I had no idea what he was talking about and it would be years before I would hear those words again.

After Calcutta, I continued on my travels to Goa with my boyfriend Tony and a group of people, including Gerard. He was French, in his early 20s and looked like the Dwarf Gimli from *The Lord of the Rings*. He disturbed me and my flesh crawled whenever he came near me. I had no idea why I didn't like him, as he seemed like a perfectly pleasant person, but I shuddered at the thought of him. About two weeks after we met, his visa was about to run out and I was incredibly relieved when it expired and he went home.

I never heard any news about Gerard until three months later when I was in Tehran in Iran. Gerard was a distant memory as I soaked up the Persian atmosphere. But several days after I arrived in the city I felt a huge shudder through my body as I sat having a lunch of kebabs and salad. My immediate reaction was, 'Gerard's here!' and I couldn't eat another thing. I've no idea where the thought came from but I recognised the feeling. There was no doubt whatsoever that he was close.

Then my logical mind took over and I told myself, 'Don't be ridiculous – he'll be back in France.' The next day I bumped into him at the Grand Bazaar, a maze of streets and traders, and Teheran's equivalent of Camden Market. At that moment I realised I had just had my first premonition. It had taken me until the age of nineteen to awaken my Instant Intuition and switch on what I now call my 'psychic antennae'.

It would be a fitting end to this part of the story to report that years later I found out Gerard was an axe murderer. Thankfully, I never saw or heard from him again after our brief and final chance meeting. I have absolutely no idea why he gave me such a bad feeling. But to be honest, it doesn't matter. It served its purpose. From that day on whenever I experienced 'a Gerard feeling', I knew it was a warning about someone or a premonition.

After 12 months, Tony and I returned to England because our money had run out. Once home, I felt so different from everyone else. It must have been the same for sailors when they left in tall ships to explore unknown waters and came back to the same people doing exactly the same things. I was less than twenty years old and suffering culture shock by returning to the UK. Gradually, I settled back into my life. I found a job doing administration for a small engineering firm on Slough Trading Estate. The whole set-up resembled the BBC sitcom *The Office*. I rented a flat in central Slough with Tony and went to the pub on Friday and Saturday nights.

But there was something different about me, thanks to what I'd learned from Vikram, although on the surface I appeared to be exactly the same. Every so often I would just 'know' something was going to happen. For example, I was sitting in the pub with a happy couple, my friends, and had a flash in my mind that they would split up. It happened six weeks later. Another time I had the same premonition with my Aunt Val and Uncle George. It was as simple as having the words 'they will split up' pop into my mind and a feeling this was 100 per cent true.

Two months later, after 25 years of marriage, my aunt and uncle divorced, which was a complete shock to everyone apart from me.

At this point in my life I had no control over my 'gift' or 'curse', depending on your perception. But I think I was able to pick up events like marriage break-ups because sadness causes a big ripple of energy and upset in people's lives. I'd developed the exercise I referred to earlier, called 'The Album'. I lay in bed and pictures appeared in my mind when I was trying to fall asleep. It was like watching a video on fast-forward and the frame would stop at a particular person. This would be the family member who was in trouble in some way. It was during this time that I recalled Vikram's words 18 months before: 'If you shut up long enough, if you still your monkey mind, you can ask and receive answers to any question.' I understood exactly what my first spiritual mentor was trying to teach me. Now, for the first time, I was starting to have some control over my psychic abilities.

....

The Album

The Album is very good for discovering information about people and situations. It's perfect because in simple terms it gives you the thumbs-up or thumbs-down about someone. I use it to test out who I should be spending time with socially, who would be a positive business contact, who I can trust. Whenever I need to find the answer to questions regarding my relationship with someone, be it business or personal, I use The Album technique.

◆ Think about a decision you need to make. It could be who to see at the weekend, who to hire and fire or even date. Don't think about any particular person – just focus on the decision and the outcome.

◆ In your mind, imagine a big red book. It's very plush with a red velvet cover and gold writing – just like a very expensive photograph album. Inside this album are pictures of everyone you have ever known, ever met, and even people you have yet to meet.

◆ Erase everything from your mind except the decision you need to make now. Keep the album in the centre of your mind and open the first page and allow the following pages to flash past you. Don't try to think about any particular person – just allow the pages to fly past as if you're flicking through very quickly.

◆ Now when you're ready, the book will suddenly slow down and stop. There in front of you will be a face. This person will be the individual who is right for the situation.

◆ You can also use this technique to choose everything from a new home to a holiday destination, car or even place of work. In the way that people will flash before your eyes, so will images representing the best course of action for you at that particular time.

....

After developing, and practising, with The Album, I realised that my gift was incredibly accurate. As time passed and my niggle disappeared, I relaxed into my craft and I craved more information on all things psychic. These days we're all falling over books on every subject imaginable and the Internet has a wealth of information – not all of it accurate, I might add. We can go to workshops and even study under the pioneers and gurus of the New Age movement. It seems odd that just over 30 years ago there was hardly any information anywhere on the esoteric arts. You had to be careful about openly discussing things like psychic phenomena and healing, let alone past-life regression or astral travel. People would assume you were weird, dangerous and probably crazy. So, I developed a double persona. By day I spent the next two years working in the office, and by night I studied every psychic book I could track down.

I was given dog-eared tomes by friends, picked up second-hand books in charity shops and occasionally had the spare cash to buy new volumes from the only occult bookshop trading at the time. Watkins Books, in Charing Cross Road, London, has been open and selling books on the esoteric since 1901 and it was a haven for someone like me – a budding psychic. It has rows and rows on everything from astrology to reincarnation, to spontaneous human combustion. Although reading is a major factor in learning, you need to practise to build your psychic 'muscles', which is why I've included exercises in every chapter of this book.

Trust your gut feeling

In his book *Blink*, Malcolm Gladwell cites dozens of examples of instant knowing. He found that people were far more accurate when they made a snap judgement than when they studied all the evidence and thought things through.

In one of his examples he talks about an art dealer, Gianfranco Becchina, who approached the J. Paul Getty Museum in California. The dealer told the museum he had a marble statue dating back to the 6th century BCE. His asking price was $10 million. The museum brought in experts, who studied the statue for months. They also looked into the documentation and history. The experts satisfied the Getty Museum, and this produced so much excitement in the art world that *The New York Times* gave it a front-page splash.

Then something strange began to happen. Several respected people 'felt' something was wrong with the statue. They couldn't explain it. Italian art historian Federico Zeri said something didn't look right with the fingernails. Then Evelyn Harrison, a world leading expert on Greek sculpture, said her first impression was great disappointment. When questioned, she said something was wrong and she didn't know what. It was just a hunch, an instinctive sense.

Some months later the former director of the Metropolitan Museum of Art in New York, Thomas Hoving, dropped in to have a look. He had developed his own method of Instant Intuition. He always made a note of the first word that came to mind. And on this occasion the word was *fresh* – hardly the word you would expect from a sculpture dated the 6th century BCE. He advised the museum to get their money back.

From this moment on, expert after expert just felt and saw something that put doubt into their mind. One art historian even described their first reaction to the sculpture as 'intuitive repulsion'. Later, the statue was found to be a fake.

Malcolm Gladwell believes that the mind has a way of taking a slither of information and discovering everything it needs to know. But if we stop and think, we cloud our judgement by bringing in our 'logic'. Trust your Instant Intuition, go with your first word and your gut reaction. It won't let you down.

Taming the monkey mind

Personally, I have spent many hours practising spiritual techniques and one of the first I learned to master was to quieten the 'monkey mind'. Again, Vikram taught me this meditation exercise in India but at the time I didn't have the patience or skill to concentrate.

'The Monkey Mind' is a wonderful exercise because it teaches you to focus your thoughts. Our minds have a tendency to jump from one thing to another. Vikram instructed me to sit quietly and focus on just one thing and one thing only. Every time my thoughts went to something else I was to steer them back to the subject in hand. At first my mind would keep wandering off, but after some practice I found I could concentrate on just one thing and exclude everything else. Even when my tummy was rumbling for food, instead of thinking, 'I'm hungry', somehow my mind would ignore this fact and stay focused. It takes practice but it's well worth it!

When your mind is still, you can connect with your intuition. And every night, after a day writing boring letters and answering the phone in the office on the industrial estate in Slough, I turned off the lights and opened the curtains so the moonlight and street lamps shone into my lounge. A single candle burned on my wooden coffee table and I sat cross-legged with my thumb touching my index finger making an 'O' shape. I'd seen people sitting like this in the ashram and when I tried the position it was indeed the best way to sit and practise meditation.

Then I would breathe in deeply and exhale slowly and begin my daily 10-minute practice. Like me, you will notice that the amount of time you can focus for builds up quickly because this is a simple exercise. One of the traditional methods for learning meditation is to focus on a flame, empty your mind and try to count up to ten.

'This is a ridiculous concept,' Vikram told me, laughing. 'If you tell a man not to think of a blue elephant he will think of a blue elephant. You put the image into his mind.' He maintained that the best way to meditate is to think of an object and to focus your whole being on exploring every aspect of it. 'This way, your mind has something to play with,' he explained with a twinkle in his eye, adding, 'Yet at the same time you are training it.' Despite the fact that he was sitting on a roadside covered in dust and didn't own a single pair of shoes, I knew these were wise words.

Daily sessions of 'The Monkey Mind' will benefit every area of your life. Although meditation has been practised for thousands of years in the East, it's only now that the health benefits are being acknowledged by the Western medical profession. Research shows that it reduces blood pressure and hypertension and it's long been recognised as a stress buster and an excellent way of reducing anxiety. Controlling your mind and your thought energy is one of the major foundation blocks that anyone wishing to train in the esoteric arts should master.

....

The Monkey Mind

◆ Put on the answering machine and tell those you live with that you need ten minutes of 'me time'.

◆ Sit in a relaxed position, cross-legged if this is comfortable. Breathe in and out deeply a few times.

◆ Think of an object – it could be an apple, a chair, even a tree. Focus your thoughts totally on this item. Visualise it clearly in your mind's eye and explore it. If it's an apple, look at the colour of the skin and the tiny imperfections. Are there any bumps? Go inside, what colour and shape are the pips? Imagine the taste and the smell.

◆ Every time your mind wanders off, let the intruding thought come in and float out as you turn back to exploring your object. You will find that you can focus on your apple for longer and longer. Your monkey mind will jump about less and your concentration will improve. In turn, this will help you undertake stronger visualisations – and as any good psychic knows, visualisation is one of the secret keys to connecting with the universe.

....

As well as meditation and visualisation, tarot cards are another good building block for psychic students. They act as a trigger and create a visual link between your intuition and your conscious mind. When I was twenty-three my best friend Terri bought me a tarot pack. Three years before, I had tried to learn the tarot and found it very hard because a traditional deck has

78 cards, all of which have different meanings. Also, there were so many different spreads and numerous interpretations for the various combinations of cards that I felt my head would pop with information overload. So I gave up. But, as I opened the new Rider–Waite pack (the most popular type of tarot pack) it felt different. I picked up the deck and knew instinctively the meaning of every card as I flicked through them, turning them over one by one as if playing a game of patience. Each card spoke to me and put pictures into my mind.

Even though it's so long ago, I can remember the first reading I did for another person because it was simple and accurate. I did a basic three-card spread for my friend Kat, and I instantly knew that the Ten of Cups showed a happy home life but with a lack of money, as represented by the Four of Coins reversed. Her third card was the page of coins. I knew immediately that she would be having a child.

Kat was adamant she would never be short of money. She said her career was her main interest and she had no intention of settling down or having a baby. Within weeks she met the love of her life and before long fell pregnant. Kat left her well-paid career to bring up her child and although money was tight, her personal life blossomed.

As well as a 'knowing' when I read the cards, sometimes a pile of words would jump into my head showing me what I needed to pass on to my client. Other times I would get a strong feeling, which was almost overwhelming, about a situation or person.

If you want to read the tarot but feel you can't connect with the pack, or have trouble remembering all the different meanings, you're trying too hard. Just let go, look at the pictures and they will tell you what you need to know about the reading.

Remember, the gypsies who invented this ancient method of divination from playing cards couldn't read and they didn't learn the skill from books. They relied on Instant Intuition.

Case study

Ellie, an accountant, attended my psychic development course then signed up for my 'Learn Tarot in a Day'. I love both of these workshops because my students learn techniques they can use immediately. Ellie was inquisitive and came on my tarot course because she wanted to learn how to use the cards to find out what was going to happen concerning her love life and career for herself and her friends.

Her first question summed up what everyone wants to know about reading the deck. 'How do you know the hidden information which doesn't appear on the cards?' I told her, 'It just pops into your head. It will just happen when you relax and let the cards speak for themselves. You won't even know you're doing it.'

Only three months later Ellie was reading for a friend of a friend and said to the rather straight-laced looking woman, 'I'm picking up that you're drinking far too much vodka. You're binge drinking and need to stop.' She didn't know the girl even drank. Apparently she was right.

When Ellie related the tale to me later I asked, 'So where did that come from? There isn't a "binge drinking vodka" tarot card.' Ellie told me matter-of-factly, 'Oh it just came into my head. I knew the information was spot on.' She had finally tapped into her Instant Intuition. Once you start practising you will notice and be able to utilise your sixth sense too. Your Instant Intuition will become stronger and your messages will become clearer. Just remember, relax, open up and don't ignore the signs.

Back to my story, two months after receiving my tarot cards as a gift, I put an advert in the local weekly newspaper. It read, 'Tarot Consultant, home visits', followed by my phone number. In the first weeks I had five clients and realised I could do this for a living. So I handed in my notice at the insurance firm, where I was now working as a rep, and set myself up as a fortune teller.

Rather like working out in a gym, my psychic abilities grew stronger the more I used them. I realised that something else was happening. I was beginning to see and feel people's energy. I took time out to feel people's vibrations. Being aware of people's 'vibes' is quite subtle but noticeable. However, there was nothing dramatic about it. With one person I simply felt tired, with another I would get a headache, and with a third I felt light-headed after being in their company for a short space of time. On the other hand, there were people who left me feeling happy and full of life.

One friend I used to meet regularly for lunch always seemed to leave me with indigestion. At first I blamed the food but then we tried different restaurants. After a while I realised there was a pattern. People who were demanding gave me a headache. It actually felt like someone had whacked me around the head. People who left me feeling light-headed usually led chaotic lives and depressed people drained my energy. I would feel as if

I wanted to crawl off somewhere and sleep for an hour or two. Lovely, warm, caring people made me feel energised – almost as if they had given me a gift.

Switching on your own psychic antennae

Have you ever noticed how some men and women are a magnet for the right people? Some of my most successful clients use their psychic antennae to great effect. They do not mix with hangers-on or dysfunctional or disloyal people who would drag them down. Instead they surround themselves with friends and associates who are warm, clever and on their side. You can use your psychic antennae to do the same and you will have wonderful people in your life. The saying goes that you're reflected by the company you keep. By having the right folk around you, you will become stronger and more confident.

Most of your important questions concerning your life will be about people, be they friends, relatives, lovers, colleagues or even your boss. Imagine being asked out on a date by an interesting man or woman, then tapping into them and feeling your energy fall through the floor. You would instantly know that this person would be wrong for you.

This simple exercise will help you to recognise and fine-tune your own psychic antennae.

Tuning In

◆ Choose five people in your life. They can be from the present or the past. I want you to pick (1) someone you adore, (2) a person you find really good fun, (3) a bore, (4) an individual who has upset you and (5) a person who has brought happiness or something good into your life.

◆ Take the first person – someone you **adore** or **love**. Picture them in your mind. Imagine talking to them. Think about all the things you've experienced with them and notice exactly how replaying these memories makes you feel. Do this for several minutes and really tap into the feelings they create when they're near you. Do you have a warm glow? Are you smiling?

Is there any particular part of your body that you're aware of during this exercise? Maybe there's a tingle in your tummy or a warm glow around your head. Maybe your shoulders have relaxed. Do you feel heavier or lighter? You need to be aware of these emotions because you will want to recognise them in the future.

Once you have identified these feelings, make a note of them. By the way, you can spend time with the person, or call them, then immediately afterwards do this exercise, and it will be even easier. You will be surprised at the number of feelings you can categorise (joy, love, relaxation – the list is endless), rather than just viewing the person as someone who makes you 'feel' good.

◆ Now focus on someone who is really **good fun**. Feel yourself smiling as you relive some of the times you have enjoyed together. Now notice where the sensations are in your body. Do you have a warm glow across your chest? Perhaps you're automatically smiling when you think of them.

Tap into the feeling and log it. In other words, make a mental note and also write down anything you're aware of regarding your emotions or feelings about this particular person. Over time you will notice more sensations, and you can add these to your notes.

◆ Now bring to mind an individual who **bores** you. Perhaps this man or woman is a work colleague or an acquaintance. Notice how you feel, how you stand or sit when you connect with them. The first time I developed, and tested, this exercise my whole body slumped, the corners of my mouth turned down and my speech became slower. I felt heavy and flat. The person I was thinking of was Ronald, the pub bore.

◆ Think of a person who has **upset you**. Many people can associate this reaction with an ex-partner, or maybe a difficult relative who has been unkind. I once had a boss who was so rude to me that for years I wanted to meet him in the street and tell him exactly what I really thought of him. When I recalled working with him my stomach dramatically tensed up and my jaw tightened. You may feel anger rising up in your throat when you do this exercise. Again, log the feelings.

◆ Finally, recall someone who is positive, a person who has brought **something good** into your life. I tried this exercise recently with one of my students, Jayne, a twenty-five-year-old fashion stylist. She smiled as she pictured her lovely boss. Her superior has backed her career and shown a great deal of faith in her abilities. As Jayne tapped into her, she broke into a broad smile and her facial features softened. Her whole body also relaxed.

....

Now your own psychic antennae are switched on, I want you to keep a track of the signals they give you. You can tune into people – note the sensations they create and slot the person into your existing categories (the bore, the good-fun person and so on). Now you can act accordingly and only spend time with people who enrich your life. This in turn creates positivity, which grows, multiplies and blossoms. After a while, using your antennae will become second nature and you will know who to talk to and who to avoid.

A top businessman and personal friend of mine has this practice down to a fine art. Everyone seems to want something from him, hoping his success will rub off on them. At parties I watch him manoeuvre away from those who are determined to talk to him but are simply takers. He calls it his 'body swerve'. Yet within minutes he will be talking to the most fascinating person in the room. Try it – you will be amazed at how much your circumstances alter for the better once you cut out the people who upset you. These types of sad souls will suck you dry and never have a good word to say about anyone or anything. Walk away and let them spiral downwards on their own. They are not going to drag you down with them.

Practice makes perfect

For the next week I want you to meet as many people as possible. Just for a split second, stop and notice your immediate feelings towards them. Here are a few examples to help build up your psychic muscles.

◆ When you pay for your petrol, notice how you feel when you speak to the cashier. Is it pleasant? Or do they bore or even upset you?

◆ When meeting a friend's boyfriend, your future mother-in-law or a new employee at work for the first time, tune into the first feeling you're aware of in connection with this person. Is this a good or a negative emotion?

◆ In a shop, smile at the person next to you in the queue and, if you can, make conversation. How do they make you feel?

◆ Now come back to your box of characters. Have you managed to find someone for each of the six categories?

If you have to spend time with people who fit into any of the negative categories – the bore, the person who upsets you (you may have to work with them) – don't worry. In the next chapter I will teach you how to protect yourself psychically using a simple exercise that stops people from draining your energy. You can follow this simple protection visualisation every morning even if you don't think you need a psychic shield, just for good measure. It will keep you protected from people who unconsciously or consciously want to harm you. Remember, your energy is precious so don't give it away unless it's to someone you love or who deserves it.

Golden handshake

Robert, the MD of one of the UK's biggest financial institutions, has perfected his own personal psychic antennae. And his method works instantly. I actually met him at a party and after learning I was a professional psychic, Robert confided, 'As soon as I shake a person's hand I can tell if they're right for me to employ. At first I didn't trust such a snap judgement, but I've learned to my cost that this works better than any interview.'

The next stage in the development of your Instant Intuition is to integrate this way of being into your everyday life. It might be an idea to start your own spiritual journal to keep a record of your thoughts and reflections as you do the exercises that follow. I promise it will make interesting reading later.

CHAPTER 2
Developing Your Everyday Intuition

My partner Tony and I decided to move from central Slough when I became pregnant. I was desperate for more space now we were going to be a family, so I put our names down for a council house. My psychic skills even helped me to find our new home. How? As I sat in the council office going through the options of what was available, the housing officer mentioned there was a large property free in Mead Avenue, in Langley, Slough. As soon as he started talking about the house I felt a tingle down my spine.

'I'll take it,' I replied.

'But you haven't seen it yet,' he said, surprised.

It didn't matter. I knew the house was right for us because a tingle for me was a positive sign. On paper it was perfect – a large semidetached property built in 1919. I was amazed no-one else had snapped it up. But I had no idea Mead Avenue was in a notorious area. Heavily pregnant, I went to view our new home for the first time the following morning. As I got off the bus and turned the corner, I couldn't believe my eyes – halfway up the road were two women fighting in the street. Despite this unexpected greeting party, I glanced at the house and knew it was where I was meant to put down roots. We moved in when Lucy was six days old and I lived there for the next 20 years and loved every minute of it.

I felt safe bringing my children up in the street. We all kept an eye on each other's offspring, did our neighbours' shopping and moaned over cups of tea – or something stronger. Not surprisingly in such a close-knit community, word spread that I was a fortune teller. So as well as people from central Slough, a steady stream of new folk came knocking at my door wanting readings. Unfortunately, hardly any clients paid me because money was tight for everyone and I was often given cigarettes, alcohol and even half-bags of coal as a thank you.

Despite the lack of hard cash, I couldn't turn people away. My strength as a reader, which I like to think I still possess, was in understanding people's problems. I had working girls, villains, people hiding from partners, battered wives – they knew they could tell me they were having an affair and the information never left the room. The consultation was between them, me and the tarot. It was not my job to judge anyone.

Liberty takers

As well as the polite villains and my sweet regulars, there were also some big liberty takers. They would phone me at all hours of the day and night, turn up on my doorstep and claim to have no money. I was a soft touch and I let them walk all over me. Some clients marched in with half a dozen kids, who wrecked my house while their mum sat for hours asking questions about whether their husbands would go to prison or if their lovers would leave their wives. Then they would throw me a small amount of money.

The phone also rang constantly and I was often exhausted and totally fed up. Over the next year, I had more and more incidences of clients turning up without warning and giving me a sob story about having no money even though they had expensive cars and smart clothes. I found it hard to turn them away. I knew I was a mug but I felt as if it was my duty to help anyone and everyone with their problems. It seemed wrong to have insight and not use it. This was my problem – I had an inability to create boundaries in my psychic work.

While I was being drained by some clients, the upside was that the sheer numbers of people meant I was using my intuition many times a day in my readings. It was like accelerated learning! Often I received flashes of information, which came in words, and the more I used my psychic gifts the more my skills became stronger and more accurate. I even began to see mini-movies in my consciousness, which played like old black-and-white films, and I was able to pass on the information. I saw couples standing at the altar getting married, people moving into new homes, new babies being cuddled and snapshots of important events.

Unfortunately, as quickly as my spiritual self grew, my physical and emotional being went downhill. I suffered with violent stomach pains which left me gasping for breath, and constant headaches which meant I had to lie in a darkened room. Often, I couldn't sleep. My lifestyle didn't help matters. I was so stressed, I couldn't seem to block out people's problems, and my ever-growing list of clients was draining the life out of me. But, then, I knew nothing about protecting myself. Yes I had read the spiritual books, including *Castaneda*, which I told you about in Chapter 1, but they were philosophical or full of complicated explanations of astrology and didn't cover the nitty-gritty of things like opening up and closing down. There were no psychic-development manuals then, and no respectable high street bookshop had a mind, body and spirit section. Such a thing just didn't exist.

Now I realise I was picking up negativity from certain clients because I was totally open psychically. I knew certain people left me tired after readings – people I now call psychic vampires – but I didn't know they were responsible for the headaches, insomnia and stomach pains that haunted me. Also, some days I was in the supermarket and suddenly I would have an over-whelming feeling of sadness, worry or even joy. I realise now that I was also picking up on the energies around me, but back then I thought it was my own mixed-up emotions. I was having trouble separating my life from those of my clients. I remember once just sitting on the bus and having this overwhelming urge to cry. I couldn't explain why I felt tearful – that was the worrying part of it all. My emotional state was putting a strain on me. Plus, the constant interruption to home life from my clients was making me feel as if I never switched off from my work.

However, fate brings people our way just when we need them. The first time I spoke to Lucy was on the phone. She had been given my number by an acquaintance and asked, 'Do you do home visits? I'd love a reading but I've broken my foot and I can't drive.' I liked the sound of her voice and I agreed to go and see her the next week at her house, which was only 20 minutes away by car.

During the reading she nodded as I went through the cards and told her what I was picking up. I could see she had a knowledge of the esoteric shown by the appearance of the High Priestess card. I asked her, 'What do you do?' She told me, 'The same as you. I didn't want to say before, but I'm a clairvoyant and that was a very good reading. Thank you. Now I have something to tell you.' I was surprised but listened. 'Don't let people take liberties,' she said. 'They'll call all hours of the day and night. Put your foot down, get a separate phone line, only see people by appointment.' She could see from the look on my face I knew exactly what she was talking about and that I needed the advice. I drove home with a firm resolution to be more assertive.

I began to try and keep set times with clients but it was difficult. People can be pushy and some clients totally ignored me when I told them they would need to make a proper appointment. Others even turned quite nasty. The negative clients were dragging me down and I was shattered, pale, thin, not eating properly and drinking endless cups of sugary tea to keep me going. My stomach pains were now coming daily and I had at least one migraine a week. I needed help.

My doctor was sympathetic but so busy he only had time to offer me medication. I didn't need drugs. I was just under pressure and open psychically, but again, I wasn't aware of this at the time. I didn't know where to go for help. My partner was working away most of the time, so I felt very alone. I had answers for my clients and neighbours but I didn't have any for myself. I was anxious about my health. Some nights as I lay in bed my whole body buzzed with worry, yet I didn't know why. I knew I wasn't depressed because some days I was full of life and happiness. So what exactly was wrong with me?

A friend suggested I see a therapist called Greta Gill. I had heard about this 'amazing woman' from other people too, who all told me the same thing, 'Greta has the answers to everything.' By the time I arrived on Greta's doorstep I was twenty-eight years old.

Strictly speaking, I didn't land on Greta's doorstep because she didn't have one. She lived on a narrowboat on the Thames in Wraysbury, Surrey, alongside a piece of land she owned directly opposite her mooring. The small field was home to a comfortable log cabin which she used for her sessions, along with her boat. Inside, the cabin housed two comfy chairs, a portable heater and a few books. Crystals hung in the window and outside there was a bench positioned to catch the sun.

Greta herself was in her 50s and had the biggest smile I had ever seen. Nothing ever rattled her. She was tiny but filled any room that she entered and everyone who knew Greta loved her. When we first met, I had seen an array of healers, herbalists and counsellors. You name it, I tried it, but still my problems persisted. Counsellors said very little and their sessions consisted of them nodding a great deal and asking, 'So, how have you been feeling this week?' Greta was different. Although she was a fully trained psychotherapist, social worker, counsellor and healer, she practised a unique form of treatment that she had developed called *psycho-spiritual reorientation therapy*. She could instinctively pinpoint exactly what you were feeling and what your problem was with very little exchange.

She also expressed an opinion that was in sharp contrast with the mute counsellors I had visited. Greta would walk around the boat or her cabin waving her arms, then suddenly would stop, look at me, then tell me exactly what I needed to know. She was always right and one of the most remarkable people I have ever met.

In our first session, she asked me briefly about my daily life and I told her about my children and mentioned that I read tarot cards. Greta immediately asked me, 'When you do a reading, how do you protect yourself?'

I had no idea what she meant and told her, 'I don't do anything to protect myself.'

Greta revealed, 'You're like a radio receiver picking up other people's emotions in your everyday life.' She explained this was why I was having such mood swings and headaches and told me how experienced clairvoyants shut down to block off this interference. With her help I learned how to protect myself. Greta showed me how to open up and close down and gave me the basics of psychic protection.

Importantly, these simple exercises helped me to train myself to switch on when I worked with the cards and switch off when I put them down. This meant I was no longer being bombarded with information, people's feelings and picking up any loose astral energy. It's imperative if you are working in this field that you learn to open up and close down and how to protect yourself. The methods outlined next are simple and straightforward.

This opening-up exercise is an easy way of tapping into your psychic mind and allowing your intuition to flow. There are many complicated books just on the topic of opening up, closing down and psychic protection but Greta boiled down these techniques to a few simple steps. I've used these routines for over 25 years and they work.

You can do this three-step exercise for switching on your Instant Intuition anywhere and at any time. Think of it as turbo-boosting your psychic powers, but remember to shut down afterwards using the exercise that follows.

Get into a routine of opening up before you do anything of a spiritual nature and think of it as one half. The other half is the closing-down exercise. Don't skip this part of the book. If you do, you'll be like those people who get into a car, have a few lessons, and then think they are ready for their driving test.

....

Opening Up

This is a three step-process.

1. Sit or stand and allow your body to loosen. Feel the muscles around your eyes and mouth relax and allow yourself a slight smile. Feel your shoulders coming down and any tension in your back or neck easing. Now feel the relaxing feeling flowing up and down your body.

2. Allow your breathing to deepen and become even and flowing comfortably. Allow any thoughts that come into your mind to float away for this short time. You do not need them for a little while.

3. Now imagine a beautiful white light shining down from the universe. See it flowing right into the top of your head, flowing down, shooting through every limb and connecting you to the universal energy that knows everything. Feel the energy connect you and fill you with brilliant white light, love and positive energy. Really use your imagination and visualise a sparkling, shimmering light flowing down towards you. The more vivid you make it the better. I like to visualise it like a high-powered shower raining down silvery white energy that flows into the top of my head and then flows to every cell of my body. I then imagine it flowing beyond my body and giving my whole aura a shimmering glow. Try it. It will give you a feeling of peace and calmness.

A quick word about the white light. This feels different for everyone who uses it. You may experience a little tingle or even a slight shiver. You may feel cool, or be aware of a sensation like a soft breeze. You are unique and will have your own way of being aware of the white light. For you it may feel warm or, as one of my students said, 'a little zing'. It may be subtle, but if you relax you will be aware of it and you will know what to expect in future.

Creative visualisation

In the above exercise, when you imagine the white light you're actually using visualisation, which is a bit like daydreaming. However, with visualisation the images in your mind are focused and you are in control; in daydreaming you allow your mind to wander. With visualisation there is a spiritual outcome and throughout this book you will learn many techniques that use the simple power of visualisation – or 'mind power', as I like to sometimes call it.

'Lucky people make effective decisions by listening to their intuition.'

Professor Richard Wiseman, author of *The Luck Factor*

Often, people tell me they can't visualise. I ask them, 'What's the colour of your front door? Where's your letterbox?' As they reply, 'Red, the letterbox is at the bottom of the door,' I tell them, 'You've just visualised your front door. You wouldn't be able to answer the question if you couldn't visualise.'

People have misconceptions about what visualisation is. They think that if they visualise a tree it will be the same as standing in front of a tree and looking at it. I then tell them, 'Don't think of a green steam train.' Of course, as soon as I say it they think of a green steam train. The image will be in their mind's eye. Just for a moment, think of a round ball. Now make it red, now shiny. Watch it bounce. Make it square, now blue, make it a box. Your mind will automatically build these images, which shows that anyone can visualise images, and the more you do so the more you will strengthen the right side of your brain.

People who use their right side – or right *hemisphere* – of their brain tend to be more psychic because that's the side we use when we are using our intuition. So if you are creative or work in a caring profession, you are more likely to be psychic. More logical individuals who use the left side of their brain, such as accountants and scientists, find it harder to visualise, but by using the above exercise you will soon strengthen your psychic mind. And the more you use it the stronger it gets.

Closing Down

◆ Whenever you finish any of the psychic exercises above, you will need to close down afterwards. This has the benefit of bringing you back down to earth. Otherwise you could feel a little light headed or 'away with the fairies' as my gran used to say!

◆ Sit quietly for a few moments then breathe deeply. As you breathe in, feel your body and mind being energised and cleansed. Then as you breathe out, release any residue you may have picked up, especially if you have been tuning in to or for someone else. If they are depressed, angry or have any other negative feelings, you will be left with some of their emotions around you. This exercise will clean it all away.

◆ Breathe in and out at least five times. Breathe in cleaning energy and breathe out anything you need to release.

◆ Now imagine you are sitting under a shower. This particular shower is very special. Imagine a silvery white sprinkle coming from the shower and washing over you, just like water cleansing and clearing you. You may even feel a little tingle as it works its magic.

....

In that first session with Greta, after telling me about surrounding myself with white light, she then gave me the best piece of advice I've ever received on protection. She said, 'If you are connected to the universe and your spirit guides, they will protect you.' My mentor also added, 'The best protection you can have is to have a true and honest heart.' I know she is right. An honest and caring heart brings in the light of love and protection. As soon as you get into murky shades of grey your energy drops. You leave yourself wide open to bad energy and the lower astral plane and psychic attack, and this can result in illness, feelings of lethargy and downright bad luck. As with everything in the universe and beyond, there is good and bad. The spirit world is no different. There are energies, entities and spirits out there that are not nice and can even be downright unfriendly or hostile. As long as you protect yourself properly you will probably never have a problem. The key is not to focus on them and to have a clear conscious and positive purpose — that way they will not be drawn to you.

Seeing the light

There are many techniques, but I find simply putting a pure white light around yourself and anyone you want to protect does the job. What follows is the method Greta taught me and, again, this uses visualisation. By using your psychic protection each and every day you will be increasing your spiritual connection and strengthening your psychic abilities.

By surrounding yourself with white light you build a protective shield around your spiritual body so that, in your everyday life, you will repel negative people and attract good souls who will be drawn to your sparkling aura. Use the white light every day and not only will it guard you against negativity, but it will also draw positive situations towards you.

Psychic Protection

1. Imagine the white light pouring down from the universe and totally surrounding you. Feel that the white light is cleansing and nothing bad can penetrate it. See and sense the white light surrounding you like a force field. Make it as real as you can imagine.

2. Watch it fill your entire aura and beyond, and in your mind's eye watch anything negative bounce off and away into the distance. Don't worry if at first you can't see it in your mind's eye. Instead, try holding a photograph of yourself and imagine a white light surrounding your image. This will give you a feeling of wellbeing and after a while you will have no need to use the photograph. With practice you will be able to surround yourself with white light instantly.

   Once you manage to get a strong flow of white light you can increase the energy and allow it to fill your entire home, giving it a feeling of peace as if you were in your own sanctuary.

3. You can ask the white light for any help you need. As your white light grows, it will build a direct link to the universe. You will find that simply imagining a white light flowing to and from your head to the universe will give you the connection you want – almost as if you have a direct line to the cosmos. This request for help can be anything from clearing a headache to help paying a bill. White is purity and the highest energy of all.

All my students follow these practises and are amazed by their effectiveness. They will protect you, help you focus your mind before you begin any psychic work and are the building blocks for any spiritual work, be it looking into the future or working on an energetic level as a healer. My advice is to use these two basic exercises to build up your visualisation techniques.

Psychic vampires

Another major form of protection that you can implement into your life is to keep away from anything that could be a problem, such as a ouija board. A ouija board is like a portal between the spirit world and our reality – and having one around is like leaving a door open to the elements. Over the years I have spoken to many people who have had nasty or inappropriate messages from them. They have told me that at first the messages contain very accurate information such as someone's date of birth, or their auntie's address, but slowly the messages become more manipulative and sinister. I would therefore steer clear of this tool of contacting the spirit world.

Also keep away from people you suspect are dishonest – you don't want your energy tarnished by their lack of honesty. Why are the people we mix with so important? People who operate in a dishonest or negative way create an energy field that is draining. We all give off energy, a feeling, and some energy workers believe that these people create tentacles that stretch out and hook into you, zapping your own energy. I call these people *psychic vampires*. I first realised they existed after I'd had my eyes opened to the need for protection by Greta, because the more I used my psychic abilities, the stronger they became. I began to see and feel people's energy.

I realised that some clients had been draining the life out of me and I became convinced the more negative ones had been the cause of my health niggles – the severe headaches and exhaustion. This realisation made me vow to always protect myself before working and to open up and shut down. Like everyone else, you don't always have complete control over the people you have to mix with, so here are some tips on how to spot a psychic vampire.

Spot the psychic vampire

You will soon know if you are in the presence of a psychic vampire because:

◆ you will feel tired and drained

◆ you will find yourself doing things you really don't want to do

◆ they will talk a lot but listen very little

◆ they complain a great deal and always seem to have a long list of problems and grudges

◆ they are self-absorbed and very demanding

◆ they usually invade your body space.

Create a psychic vampire shield

Once you've spotted a psychic vampire, you'll need some tips on how to combat them.

◆ Don't face them, but stand at an angle to them – it will then be harder for them to connect and drain your energy.

◆ Keep one hand on your solar plexus (your upper abdominal area), because this will stop them draining your life force. This is a key energy point that needs protecting.

◆ Imagine you are inside a bubble, then fill it with white light.

◆ Move away from them as soon as you can and avoid them in the future.

◆ Spend as little time as possible in their company.

◆ Remember, they are very thick-skinned so gentle hints will not work – just leave.

Grounding yourself

Many people, as they begin developing their psychic powers, complain of headaches, feeling light-headed, dizzy or even exhausted. If you are experiencing any of these problems, and your doctor can't find a medical explanation, you need to ground yourself. Grounding yourself also protects you from intentional and unintentional psychic vampires. It's very simple to ground yourself and can take as little as 60 seconds. I know – I've timed it.

....

Grounding

Here is an exercise for grounding yourself.

1. Find yourself a quiet spot to relax. Close your eyes and take a few deep breaths.

2. Now imagine you are outside, standing or sitting in a peaceful meadow. At first, standing up as you do this exercise will be more effective. You may even spread your arms out like the branches of a tree. If you *can* actually stand or sit outside on grass, natural earth or on sand, then that's even better.

3. Connect with the outside, with nature. Feel the sun shining down on you. Listen to the sounds of nature, the birds and insects, and be aware of the plants and trees surrounding you.

4. Now imagine yourself becoming solid and strong and having roots like a tree. Feel yourself taking root, feel yourself reaching down into the earth. The deeper your roots go, the better. Now feel at one with the world and the whole of nature.

Some people like to ground themselves while standing up with their legs slightly apart – while others prefer to sit. Try out the two versions and see which one suits you. Once you have practised this exercise a few times, you will be just as effective sitting down, as standing up. With practice, you won't even have to shut your eyes to imagine the roots going into the ground. You may even feel the roots of the tree spreading out from the back of your legs and your bottom.

This technique will revive you instantly and will take nothing away from your psychic powers. The best psychics are very grounded.

Why ground yourself?

Everything is made up of energy, which constantly moves and flows, and it can be drained from you by a needy client if you work psychically or as a healer. Friends can also do this unintentionally if they're distressed. At times I have clients who are very distraught and, if I am not careful, I am completely wiped out when they leave. I have a technique that I use when I find this happening.

A draining client, or psychic vampire, usually uses an 'etheric tentacle' (more about this in Chapter 3), which they attach to the solar plexus. They don't know that they're doing this, but on an instinctive level they reach out, energetically, and steal your energy.

In order to 'break' their etheric tentacle away from my solar plexus I pretend I'm brushing something from my clothes around my middle. No-one has ever noticed me doing this but every single time I have felt the drain of energy stop and immediately my own high energy levels return.

Other times we lose our energy are when we are meditating. This is purely lack of experience and, as we open up to the universe, we allow our energy to leak instead of drawing in the wonderful universal energy. This is very easy to change – simply imagine a wonderful white light flowing into your crown chakra at the top of your head and filling you up with universal energy. You will feel revived and wonderful. (We'll look in more detail at chakras later. But suffice to say, for now, that they are centres of spiritual energy located at various points in your etheric body, beginning at the base of your spine and ending at your crown. See diagram on p. 118.)

In all cases, if you surround yourself with white light before doing anything of this nature, your own energy will stay with you and others will find it hard to take it from you.

Trusting the process

I began to see Greta once a fortnight and my confidence grew little by little. As I became stronger, my life became calmer, especially as I regularly began grounding myself. There was no overnight magic, just a growing awareness that I was feeling more centred and much less stressed. I began to say 'no' more too, and the strange thing was that when I adopted this new set of rules people took more notice of me and the liberty takers appeared less and less at my door.

As I juggled bringing up two children and seeing clients, I continued to visit Greta. Although I had driven Vikram mad with my constant questions, Greta was unflappable. She would gently tell me to quieten my mind (remember the 'monkey mind' we spoke of in Chapter 1?) and look within for the answers, but this was like telling a hyperactive four-year-old to sit still.

Her favourite saying was, 'Just trust the process.'

I would ask, 'What do you mean?'. Greta patiently explained that everything was working just as it should and that I was where I was meant to be at that moment in time. I would say, 'Oh great! I'm meant to have a hard life.'

She would smile and simply say, 'When you learn to trust the process it will all work out fine.'

Echoing my childhood, I would sit and try to have a premonition and I would attempt to trust the process. I would think of her words, 'The universe has a master plan for you. Let go and it will work out perfectly.' I would arrive at Greta's boat and say, 'I've been trusting the process and I still can't pay my electricity bill.'

She would say mysteriously, 'Oh, really? You have definitely trusted the universe to provide for you?'

I would reply, 'Oh, yes.' Somehow I had expected a cheque to pop through my front door signed 'The Universe'. It hadn't clicked then that I had to let go and trust, and what I needed would come. In the West, we are so conditioned to pushing for what we want that this can be a difficult concept to grasp. It certainly was for me at first.

One day, after I had been seeing Greta for about two months, I asked her, 'How can you hand your whole life over to the universe and trust every minute of the day?'

She replied, 'How else is there to live?'

Like a thunderbolt I remembered Vikram's words seven years before in Calcutta. Like Greta, I realised that he trusted 'the process'. He never worried about the past or the future. Vikram knew he was on his right path and the universe was taking care of him, which is what Greta also believed.

I told Greta about Vikram and asked her, 'How is it that you and Vikram say exactly the same things, yet you live totally different lives in totally different countries?'

She laughed and replied, 'We all get our information from the same place.'

Finally I was beginning to understand but I was still grappling with the concept of letting go.

How to trust the process

Ask for nothing – you know that the universe is bringing you your greater good.

Greta had faced her own personal crisis in 1977 in her late 40s, four years before we met, after she was involved in a horrific car crash. The accident claimed the life of her first husband and nearly killed her. She spent the next three years in and out of surgery and in plastercasts. This experience radically changed her belief system and connected Greta to her own spiritual awareness. When she talked about overcoming physical, emotional and spiritual pain, she did so with gentleness. She knew what it felt like because she had been through it all herself. She came out of the fire 'trusting the process'. Greta would tell me that I already had all the answers to my problems. 'All that you need to know is inside. You just have to stop and learn how to listen,' she would say patiently.

One day we were going to a talk in London on near-death experiences (NDEs) when we got stuck in a huge traffic jam. I fidgeted and worried and I complained that we would be late. Greta simply said, 'There's a reason. Just wait and see.' As we crept slowly along the road up ahead we could see roadworks. We inched forward until we were alongside a chap holding a stop sign. Greta looked over and said to me, 'Ah, that's the reason – that man needs to speak to me.'

I cringed as she stuck her head out of the window and said, 'Hey, how are you doing?'

He looked around and said, 'Oh, okay, I suppose.'

Greta replied, 'You've had a tough time recently.'

The man looked astonished and then he said sadly, 'I lost my wife a few months ago and it isn't getting any easier.'

Greta replied gently, 'She's just fine. Your wife is up there with my husband. He'll take care of her.'

I was amazed to see the man's face soften and fill with peace. He turned the sign around and we continued on our journey.

Stunned, I asked her, 'How did you know?' Greta just smiled.
I sighed, 'We'll miss our train now.'

She replied, 'We didn't want that one, anyway.'

When we arrived at the station our train was cancelled! I
began to think she had a charmed life. In the car I thought to
myself, 'It's all very well trusting the process when your life's in
order, but when you have upheavals and problems it's not so
easy.' Greta looked at me and just gave me one of her knowing
smiles. She was even aware of what I was thinking.

An everyday psychic

Over the course of our subsequent meetings, Greta taught me
how to be what I call 'an everyday psychic'. Greta tapped into
her intuition everywhere. In the supermarket she would hold
her pendulum over the vegetables to find which ones were fresh
– despite their deceptive appearances. She would also hover her
hand over the bonnets of cars to see which vehicle she should
buy. I saw her do this once in a car showroom and the look on
the salesman's face was hilarious!

She could even 'feel' which holiday destination would be most
suitable for her by running a finger slowly down a list of options
in a brochure. Greta told me she just knew when she had the
answer or the right information. My mentor made all her decisions using her Instant Intuition and she tapped into her psychic
instincts no matter what she was doing professionally or
personally.

To help me develop further, Greta encouraged me to read and
to listen to spiritual tapes – this was before the time of CDs.
One tape she lent me was by the mystic and visionary Stuart

Wilde and called *Free Flow*. On the tape, Wilde talked about flowing along with life and not wanting or worrying about anything, saying that everything is just how it should be at that moment. He said, 'When you are in flow, the lights are always green.'

In a nutshell, free flow means you send out to the universe the thought of what you need and then you stop pushing for it because you trust that it will be appear in your life. If it doesn't materialise, there is a reason which will become clear later. Another version of this concept is *cosmic ordering*, sometimes called *manifestation*, where you write a wish list to the universe for the help you need or what you desire. The TV personality Noel Edmonds credits this concept with revitalising his flagging career and landing him his dream job as presenter of Channel 4's *Deal Or No Deal*. However, years before Edmonds penned his wish list for a new life and hit TV show – which he says started to materialise within six months of his asking the universe for help – Wilde was telling people, 'Go with the flow.'

I began practising free flow on Greta's insistence and things fell into place. My day went from being chaotic and unpredictable to smooth. For example, I found that if I looked at my telephone and willed it to ring with clients calling me for appointments, it would ring.

In contrast, if I needed a quiet day I would imagine the phone silent and it would sit mute. At first I did wonder if it was a fluke, but the consistency with which my wishes were answered made me believe it was real. I would call the garage for a last-minute appointment and someone else would have just cancelled, which meant I didn't have to wait weeks to get my car fixed. It sounds mundane, but imagine life where luck is on your side – that's how it started to feel for me.

To be honest, at first the thought patterns associated with free flow weren't my natural state. But the technique did work and became a habit, a positive mindset. As I trusted the process, I attracted clients who treated me better, my finances began very slowly to improve, and because I was less wound up, I found the time to eat properly. I started to sleep more easily at night too. The combination of Greta's sessions and Wilde's free flow made my life not only less stressful but also less complicated. I began passing information on to other people about free flow, spreading the word that the universe provided if you asked for assistance.

I remember one incident when a young man called Peter came to see me. He was desperate. He had split up with his girlfriend, had lost his job and was living in one small room. I looked at his cards and told him, 'You're going to have a wonderful life. There's a gorgeous new girlfriend for you and you will be rich.' Every client wanted me to give them a message like this one but this was the first time I had seen such a wonderful spread. It had all the classic cards of abundance such as the Ace of Pentacles, which shows new income, followed by the Four of Pentacles, indicating that it would come easily. The spread was topped off by the King of Pentacles, indicating that Peter would be extremely successful in business.

Peter gave me a cynical look and said, 'Yeah, sure. I came here by bike – how am *I* ever going to make any money?'

I handed him the free flow tape and told him, 'Listen to this. You'll understand it.' He left and I never expected to see him again.

Around 18 months later, a black Porsche pulled up outside my house and Peter got out, walked up to the front door and knocked. As he handed me back the tape he said, 'This works. Boy, does it work!' Peter had started his own double-glazing business with a loan and soon made lots of cash. He had a gorgeous new girlfriend. How? He understood free flow and he had put it into practice. To recap, free flow means:

◆ you **let go** of worrying about the outcome and try not to fight against what is happening;

◆ you **trust** the universe and **ask for help** – and it provides.

Later, Greta showed me just how much faith she put in her own beliefs, when she had to leave her home, but by now the positive changes in my own life were enough to convince me it worked.

Go with the flow

Trusting the process means handing yourself over to a situation and having faith that things are happening as they should for you at that moment. Free flow is more interactive and dynamic and is almost the step before this act. With free flow you 'ask' the universe for an outcome, then step back and wait. You trust the process. Try these simple tips to help you link into free flow.

◆ For one day, let go of all expectations. Let go of what you want and let go of any worries or concerns.

◆ During that day, no matter what happens, do not rush.

Simply pace yourself and become aware of how frantic and stressed everyone else is acting.

◆ Stand still and watch and listen, but do not react.

◆ If things go wrong, then watch them unravel and know that is how your present reality should be unfolding.

◆ If someone wants something from you, either just give it to them or tell them no. Do not justify, argue or try to persuade.

◆ If people are upset, angry, demanding or in a mess, leave them be to learn their own lesson.

◆ Tell people as little as you can about yourself. Remain anonymous. Hold your energy within yourself, be still inside.

◆ Feel that you are walking along a road and you will reach your destination no matter what.

◆ Know that everything that happens along the way is just minor detail.

◆ Notice a feeling of peace as you connect with the natural rhythm of your life.

◆ Simply go with the flow.

Each time I saw Greta, I moved a little further along my path and a few years after my 'official' counselling with her had ceased and I was 'better' (meaning I was healthy and happy), I was still popping in to see my mentor to soak up her wisdom and teaching. Then, Greta had an upheaval of her own. Her doctor advised her that the damp atmosphere of the boat was getting into her bones, which were already weakened by the car crash. He told her she had to move away from the water or risk falling gravely ill.

I was frantic with worry. 'Where will you go?' I asked, trying to hide my panic.

She answered, 'Oh, the universe is sorting all that out for me.'

I worried that she was being naïve or in denial. Yes, the universe could provide an abundance of luck – but she needed to go and find somewhere 'real' to live, and fast, otherwise she would be homeless. Greta had no doubt whatsoever that 'something would come up'. I knew she had plenty of friends and I assumed she would go and stay with one of them.

The day before she was due to leave her narrowboat, I sat with Greta and she didn't have a care in the world as we listened to the ducks outside. Suddenly her phone rang and a lady at the other end said, 'Greta, this is such a cheek and such short notice, but I need a house sitter for three months. I leave tomorrow.' With a twinkle in her eye Greta gave me a big smile. She never said, 'I told you so.' By the way, when the lady said, 'house sitter' she was wrong. A more accurate description would be 'mansion sitter'. Greta had a country pile in two acres to live in for the next three months, rent-free with no bills. The week before she was due to leave, the lady called her again. The acquaintance asked Greta awkwardly, 'Is there any possible way you could stay on for another three months?' Her husband's work contract had been extended. Greta of course said yes. When Greta – she of the charmed life – told me the news with a straight face, I could not believe it.

I hesitate before telling you the next part of these magical events because it's so astonishing. The day before Greta was due to leave this gorgeous mansion a friend of the owner, who had an even bigger property, telephoned and said, 'I know this is a cheek and it's very short notice, but I don't suppose . . .'

Greta had done it again. She went on to spend another six months in a gorgeous home before moving into her own property later on. She trusted the process fully and the universe provided for her in return and in abundance. The whole episode was a perfect indication of everything Greta believed in and showed how the universe, the cosmos, really does look after you if you 'trust the process'. Any niggling doubts I had – which by then were small but surfaced occasionally – vanished.

The five-minute psychic

As a professional psychic, I meet so many people who say to me, 'I wish I had time to develop my intuition. But how can I fit it into my busy life?' There are two answers to this question. First, we make time for what we feel is important. Second, the days of sitting on top of a mountain contemplating your naval are well and truly over. We all have busy lives.

A lady called Julie came to my intuition workshop recently. She told me, 'I work hard all day, then I return home to my three noisy children. I don't have one moment's peace. I don't have time to waste doing complicated exercises and rituals.'

My response was, 'Exactly!' – and this is why I've developed Instant Intuition. During the workshop, I showed Julie techniques that she could practise in five-minute chunks throughout the day without feeling as if she had to 'make time'. You can try these techniques too. Before you know it you'll be tapping into your intuition instinctively exactly when you need to throughout the day.

As I have my breakfast, I build up a picture in my mind of my front door and I imagine the letterbox opening and envelopes dropping onto the doormat. I focus and see what letters have arrived. I will think to myself, 'Oh, the gas bill's come' or, 'Lovely, a letter from my aunt'.

If I'm meeting a friend for lunch I will focus and try to imagine what they will be wearing and what they will order to eat. You can use the same exercise for people you don't know or someone who is only an acquaintance. If I'm seeing clients I will try to imagine what they look like and very often they are exactly how I picture them. Just recently a young man called Kingsley visited me. As soon as he walked through the door I said to him, 'You know, you have a great future as a psychic yourself.' He was astonished but by tapping into him before he arrived I could feel he was special and very gifted.

There are three different routes I can take from my home to my office in Bray, Berkshire. As I start my car, I build a picture of the journey in my mind. As I do this quick exercise I will feel compelled to travel a certain way. Often I don't know why I want to avoid one road and not another but I trust my Instant Intuition. Some days I hear later that there were problems on the route I've avoided. I admit that occasionally there are days when I rush off and don't bother to tap into my gut feelings. On these rare occasions I realise that I've taken more notice of a radio report. Or I have listened to logic, which has told me something like, 'It's Ascot races week, the motorway will be jam-packed, go on the A roads.' My logical mind has made me dismiss the motorway, believing that it will be overly busy, when in fact I am leaving at a time that wouldn't clash with the race traffic.

I use my Instant Intuition all day, every day, and there is nothing I do that you can't do. The more you use these techniques, the better you will become at tapping into your Instant Intuition – which for me is now so strong that I trust it above everything else.

Case study

Jamie attended one of my workshops. He told me, 'I don't think I'm very psychic somehow. I'm a practical person. I work with my hands.' He didn't have any recollection of ever having had an incident where he had used his intuition, although I suspected he had without realising it.

It is surprising how often people will say they are not intuitive yet you will hear them say things like, 'Something doesn't feel right about this.' When you ask them why they have this feeling they have no idea.

Some months later Jamie contacted me and told me that his intuition saved his life. He told me: 'I suppose I had been using my gut feelings but I was unaware of it until a concrete block narrowly missed my head.'

Jamie had been working on a tall building. It had floor and scaffolding but no walls. The floors were being built out of concrete blocks. Jamie said, 'You can imagine the noise with 30 men all hammering and banging but for some reason I suddenly shuddered and looked up to see a concrete block flying towards my head. I jumped back and as it missed me by an inch I actually felt a whoosh of air.

'Working below was my brother-in-law. I screamed to him and he also jumped out of the way. Somehow my intuition saved both of us from getting our heads smashed to bits.'

For all of us there are times when we ignore the niggle or gut feeling. If you do ignore a sign, make a mental note when you realise your logical mind was wrong. It will help strengthen your confidence in your abilities the next time you doubt yourself or listen to other people who try to push you into things that go against your instincts. Remember when someone said, 'Let's go to the beach' or 'Why don't we go into town tonight to that new club?' and you had a sinking feeling? Despite having a gut reaction you went against it and it was a disaster. Remember those incidents the next time you have twinge and your gut reaction tells you not to do something. Go with your Instant Intuition and not the response from your logical mind.

Just a hunch

In March 2006, a drug-testing scandal hit the UK when six human guinea pigs reacted badly to a trial drug. In one case, a man's head swelled to three times its normal size within hours of his first injection of TGN1412 – medication being developed to fight rheumatoid arthritis, leukaemia and multiple sclerosis.

But Tom Edwards, who was 21, had a lucky escape. He turned down £1,100 to take part because of a hunch that it didn't feel right. At the time he was quoted widely in the UK's national press saying, 'Something told me to be suspicious about it. It seemed a bit haphazard. It's not really like me to turn down £1,100 but I wasn't comfortable doing it.'

Picking up subtle vibrations and energies

As well as trusting your gut reaction, a major part of intuition is picking up on subtle vibrations and energies. Gut reaction is the immediate response. It's a yes or no about a situation, person or decision. Picking up vibrations is a step up from gut reaction because you are tuning in and gleaning much more information about the situation, person or decision. When you can pick up vibrations you will not only know whether it's a yes or no, but you'll also know why, and all the detail that goes with it.

In my psychic-development workshops I do an exercise to help my students pick up vibrations, or what many psychics call *reading energy*. I ask someone unknown to the group to wear some bangles for a day. They then put them into a sealed envelope, which I open and tip out onto the table. I then ask the group to pick up a bangle and write down any impressions they pick up. They are not to try to guess the information but simply jot down what pops into their heads. You would expect this exercise to be a bit hit or miss because most of the group have had very little to do with developing their intuition. But the results are always remarkable, especially on my last two workshops. For one exercise three students wrote, 'This is a lady, she is big, blonde.' One person said, 'The woman has daughters.'

Three people said, 'She has recently split up with her boyfriend.' Two people believed her work was connected to flowers and one workshop participant mentioned a cottage.

The only new information for me was the part about the cottage. But when I relayed this back to the lady she told me she had just spent the weekend away in a cottage and that was exactly where she was when we were holding the workshop. She is big, blonde, has daughters and has just split up with her boyfriend and works as a florist.

On the next workshop the students held the bangles and said, 'A dark-haired girl, with foreign blood', and also wrote that she has a 'fair-haired boyfriend'. They picked up that she had been arguing with her partner and that she is very creative and a healer. The woman in questions is Italian and has a blond boyfriend, and they just had an argument before she took off the bangles. She is also a beautician and a wonderful healer. My psychic students couldn't have been more spot-on – and, remember, they were all novices. I use the same technique, picking up vibrations – or *psychometry*, to use the proper name – regularly with my clients. But you don't have to be a professional clairvoyant to utilise the skill, as my workshops demonstrate.

One of my past students, Claire, recently sent me an email asking how she could find out about a chap at work. She didn't want to make a fool of herself by asking him on a date, so she contacted me to find out what she could do. They had exchanged a few flirty emails but he seemed a little on the shy side. This is so easy, anyone can do it. I told her to go and borrow his pen. This would carry his vibrations. Once back at her desk with his highlighter, Claire focused and remembered to take the first impressions. She immediately picked up images of lots of different women whom she worked with in the same office. At first she assumed she had made a mistake. I told her to go back and trust her Instant Intuition. As you begin to 'feel' people's vibrations you will soon know if someone is just flighty or insincere. Claire tried again and still the faces of her colleagues came to her. She had the impression he was flirting with them all.

Claire telephoned me and said, 'Anne, I've done something very naughty. When he was at lunch I peeped at his emails. I know it's wrong but I really wanted to know if my gut feelings were spot-on. Can you believe it? He's quietly flirting with half the women in the building. Even the ones who are married. What a cheek! And thank God I didn't ask him out!'

Another of my psychic students asked me if she could find out how her boyfriend really felt about her. Once a month she would look after his house and cat while he worked away. She felt embarrassed to tell us she had snooped through everything trying to find a clue. She looked for a diary or something where she might have received a mention. She listened to old answerphone messages. But there wasn't a clue in sight.

I told her that if she was staying there it gave her a wonderful opportunity to 'feel' his energy and to pick up his vibrations. She could sleep in his bed and allow her dreams to connect their energy. I told her, 'Why not put on a jumper that he's worn and stick his socks on and just tap into him?' Later Jenny phoned me to say, 'Oh, dear, I cut it fine timewise and as he walked through the door I was sitting there wearing his giant jumper with my tiny feet in his large boots. He looked at me as if I was mad. I just weakly said, "I'm cold." It was quite a warm day.'

But she did connect with his energy and she could feel he really cared for her but didn't want to rush things in case it spoiled their relationship. She had the feeling he had behaved this way in the past and things had gone wrong. This time he was determined to get it right. Luckily, this incident didn't put him off too much and a short time later he proposed. She's never told him why she was wearing his very large boots on a summer's day!

The simple exercises in this book are the first steps that will help you to strengthen your own psychic muscles. They will get you into the habit of tapping into your Instant Intuition every day and picking up on the subtle vibrations around you. Before long, you will be automatically utilising your natural psychic skills and they will become second nature.

Like Greta, I now use my own skills every single part of my day. I go to a lot of social events and often my friends are amazed when I suddenly leave. I know when 'the party's over' even before it's started to wind down because I can tune into what is going on around me, in terms of psychic energy. Every time, just after I've said my goodbyes to the host, there will be a disagreement or something happens and the party atmosphere evaporates. It's important that you learn to trust this intuitive feeling and not let logic stand in the way. On occasions I've been at a bash and I've been really enjoying myself. The last thing I've wanted to do is leave but when I get the 'nudge' – which, by the way, is a sudden feeling and thought that I should leave – it comes from nowhere and I listen to it.

If I'm visiting someone's house for the first time I will try to visualise what it's like inside. I tap in and see the colour of the carpet and walls and the type of sofa – just for practice and to keep my psychic skills razor sharp. While some of the techniques I've taught you so far may sound as if I'm playing a game, this game will change your life. It will alert you to what you need to know and it will give you the edge in personal and business matters. After a while you will do it automatically and it will take you just seconds. You can use this skill to answer life's important questions concerning everything from choosing the right property to finding the best career for your talents.

But there's no doubt that one of life's most important questions is, 'Is this person right for me?' No doubt there are many other issues such as 'Will it last?' and even 'Will we have a secure future together?', which may run through your mind when you meet someone new or hit a sticky patch with your current partner. A high percentage of the women and men who visit me for a reading want to find out about their love life. If you have love, you have everything, and I have been asked numerous times, 'How do you know when you've met the one?' This is a question I have pondered.

There is only ever one answer – you can't go by your feelings. Who hasn't been in love with someone who is wrong for them? Who hasn't been out with the perfect mate who professes undying love, steals your heart and then later dumps you? The only truly accurate way of knowing who is 'the one' is that when you're with them you become greater, stronger, happier and more confident. In other words, your energy rises. When you are with the wrong person you lose part of yourself. People notice and tell you, 'You've lost your sparkle.' This reaction is all to do with energy. You need to know who builds you up and who drags you down.

The psychic-antennae technique in Chapter 1 should give you a quick answer to this question. But if you want detailed information, such as what the other person's thinking about you, you need to be able to delve into someone's feelings. The next stage of developing your Instant Intuition is EET (etheric energy technique), which takes the tools you've learned so far one stage further. EET lets you tap into a chosen person's thoughts and emotions, no matter where they are in the world. This is a priceless gift that will change your life. Use it wisely.

CHAPTER 3
Tapping into Emotions and Thoughts

I've been teaching the Etheric Energy Technique for the past ten years. The methods I'm going to reveal in this chapter will enable you to gain answers to life's important questions because this technique allows you to tap into another person's inner thoughts and emotions. Using your own energy field, you can instantly 'feel' another person's response to any question, which can save you time and effort in all areas of your life.

Even though this sounds like something the hero would do in a sci-fi blockbuster, it is real and it can be done. You can reach across continents to tap into someone's mind – even penetrating the thoughts of guarded and difficult people. You can discover what someone really thinks about you and look at yourself through their eyes.

But let's not run before we can walk! Although EET is simple and quick to do, it is advanced and you need to learn how to 'sense' energy before you try it. There are a number of ways you can connect with energy, which is what I'm now going to teach you. If you grasp these methods first, your EET will be more successful and in the long run you will have better results all round.

Sensing energy

I saw my first aura over 20 years ago when I went on a group meditation night. I was meditating as normal when I opened my eyes out of curiosity to see what everyone else was doing. I was astounded to see huge bright colours surrounding each of them. The girl who facilitated the workshop had the most amazing aura. Greta had told me that the aura was 'an energy field around people which manifests in colours. These colours hold the secrets about a person's spiritual, emotional and physical wellbeing for those that can see them.'

And here I was, looking at swirling colours pulsing around the girl, which stretched 60 centimetres (about two feet) around her body. The girl's aura was brown and gold with bands that spread out around her head and looked exactly like the stripes found on a pharaoh's sarcophagus. Later I discovered that the pictures on the mummy's coffin, and effigies in the temples of the various gods, were created to represent their auras. Now that I had seen it for myself, I could see the likeness of the aura and the Egyptian coffins.

Another girl, Shelley, an astrologer, dazzled me with a shining aura of turquoise and pink. It was beautiful. It looked like puffy little clouds. All around me I could see swirling colours that manifested in different ways. Some were spiky and were just at the front, others were in rays and some of the auras even intermingled. There was a mother and her nine-year-old son in the group and I was amazed to see that their aura of similar colours merged and swirled as one.

After the meditation we sat and had tea and chatted. I expected someone to say, 'Wow, did you see the colours?' It really was like watching the northern lights in your living room. But not a soul mentioned the beautiful spectacle. I realised I had been the only one to see the colours.

A few weeks after this experience, I went to the Mind, Body and Spirit (MBS) Festival in London. As people queued for their turn to have their auras photographed (more on this later), I studied them. I couldn't see their auras that day but I could feel them. (As I explain later in this chapter, not all psychics 'see' – some pick up vibrations through feelings. In the Appendix, at the back of the book, you can do the quiz to find out what type of psychic you are and what your particular spiritual strengths are.) I hovered around as people collected their pictures and peeped over their shoulders. They probably wondered who the strange and nosy lady was but I didn't care because, sure enough, the colours I felt were correct. I had my own aura photographed and after ten minutes I was given my photograph by an 'aura expert'. He told me what the colours represented regarding my spiritual, physical and mental being. I was thrilled to see that my aura was white, pink, yellow, lilac and purple. Apparently, this meant I was 'kind, psychic and logical with a good brain'. I was enthralled. For me, discovering this new gift of feeling the aura was like finding a new planet.

Actually being able to feel the aura at the MBS festival, and having already seen it surrounding people at the meditation group, was all the proof that I needed to believe it existed. Both experiences gave me confidence and made me realise that my ambition of developing psychic abilities hadn't been in vain. All the years of having friends, acquaintances and certain family members tell me that I was odd, or pull faces behind my back, had been worthwhile because now I had some ammunition. I had concrete evidence, a real experience, which they couldn't argue about with me or dismiss as fantasy. I felt I could now be more open about my spiritual path and my experiences and it was a real turning point in my life.

The jolly green giant

Years after I had my aura photographed I spotted a sign saying AURA PHOTOGRAPHY at a psychic fair in Berkshire. I was curious to know whether my aura had changed over time. It was a little more basic than the big booth at the Mind, Body and Spirit Festival but I thought I would give it a go. The man offering the readings told me to look into a camera so that he could take my picture, then the computer would process the image and print out the details. I patiently waited for my image to appear and as the machine spat it out I was stunned to see I looked like the jolly green giant. 'Your aura's green,' he told me. 'You're a quiet and peaceful person that loves being isolated and at one with nature.'

I had to stop myself from laughing, 'Umm, not really,' I replied. 'I prefer cities to the wild outdoors and nobody who knows me well would describe me as peaceful.' He insisted the aura was a true representation of me. At that moment I noticed a number of lights flashing on his computer. I looked over and saw beneath each flashing light a sign saying all the other colours had run out. Only green was left! Even as I pointed this out to the chap he still insisted it was a true representation and carried on taking people's money.

Not to be put off, a short time later as I walked along Hastings seafront, I spotted a machine saying, HAVE YOUR AURA PHOTOGRAPHED

HERE FOR £1. 'What a bargain!' I thought. I stood in front of the machine and placed my one-pound coin in the slot. This time a bright red picture of me appeared and below it said, 'You are angry.' Funnily enough, my friends who were with me who also put money in the machine that day were bright red and also angry.

The human energy field

These days most people have heard of the aura, the Human Energy Field (HEF) that surrounds our bodies. In fact, there has been a wealth of research actually proving its existence. The California Institute for Human Science (CIHS) has been conducting studies into ki-energy and its president, Dr Hiroshi Motoyama, has even had a paper published outlining practical exercises which boost the HEF. The Institute of Religion and Psychology in Tokyo is also pioneering experiments to study spiritual energy which include testing the chakras and meridians to understand how these affect health and the mind.

One of the first health professionals to explore the concept of the HEF was the Viennese doctor Franz Anton Mesmer, the founder of modern hypnotism, who became convinced that an electromagnetic field surrounded the human body. He developed his ideas in the 1800s and thought the energy was made up of a fluid substance. Mesmer also believed that it could affect another person. By the middle of the 19th century, Count Von Reichenbach had spent 30 years undertaking studies into HEF. He called it the *odic field*. He produced some wonderful results, in which the odic field could be conducted through a wire, and was probably the first to show scientific evidence of its existence. He found that the odic field responded to certain influences such as air current – sometimes it behaved like a gas, other times like a light wave.

Walter Kilner, from St Thomas's Hospital, London, found that he could see the human energy field by looking though a glass screen stained with dicyanin dye – he saw a glow around human bodies. In 1965, he published his work in a book called *The Human Aura*, in which he stated that each person's aura was different and was affected by their mental, emotional and physical state. Meanwhile, scientists in Russia had been carrying out their own experiments since 1939. Semyon Davidovich Kirlian and his wife Valentina accidentally discovered a flash of energy between an electrotherapy machine and a patient. They developed the procedure until they could actually see a hand as luminous, flashing, sparkling and glowing. This where the term *Kirlian photography* originated. They could also detect illness in a patient long before it showed in the body. The Kirlian photographs of someone who was sick would show irregularities in the person's aura. Sometimes dark or dull patches appeared, which would not be present in the HEF of a healthy person.

Since the 1960s, extensive research in Russia has actually broken down this energy field and discovered what it is made of. They've called it bioplasma. Dr Victor Inyushin at Kazakh University believed this to be a fifth state, the original four being solids, liquids, gases and plasma. Today there is a wealth of research into the human energy field. For instance, Charles Panati in his book *Supersenses* mentions that Dr Thelma Moss was working with Kirlian photography in Russia in the 1970s. She returned to America and built her own device, which she later used to photograph the fingertips of two people with their hands almost touching and found two interesting results. 'In some cases,' she says, 'the energy fields attract each other, and in other cases they push each other away, just like a magnet.' Moss said, 'My guess is this is why some people like each other instinctively when shaking hands. You can call it good vibes and bad vibes.'

Working with your own energy

As you become aware of your own aura and its own vibration you will become conscious of the more subtle part – the etheric. The more conscious you become of the etheric, the more you will be able to use Etheric Energy Technique. You will become aware of how everything is made up of energy. In the UK over the past 20 years, the biologist Dr Harry Oldfield has developed two innovative systems that measure and treat the subtle fields of energy around living things. The first builds on studies of the scientist's work with Kirlian photography and is called the *electro-scanning method* or ESM. Oldfield says he can obtain a three-dimensional reference field around the body using ESM.

The second of Oldfield's inventions is a camera, which he calls a PIP (*polycontrast interference photography*) scanner. It provides a real-time three-dimensional image of the human energy field – or that of any living thing. PIP records light-interference patterns (how ambient light interacts with subtle energy fields) and can even project your moving colourful aura onto a screen. Oldfield also believes PIP shows up the body's etheric template. This can be seen in his phantom leaf and phantom limb pictures using this method, which can be found in his book *Invisible Universe*.

If you ever have your aura photographed, you will immediately be struck by its bright colours, but also look at the more subtle energy surrounding it. It usually shows up as grey or a silvery shimmer. This is what I refer to as *etheric energy*.

In my workshops I teach people how to *feel* the aura first before we go on to learning how to see it. Later, my students learn how to tap into someone's energy field using EET. I believe everybody can feel and see auras. You just have to let go and tap into your inner knowing – remember, many psychics don't actually see with their eyes but with their mind. The information comes to them in flashes or pictures within their consciousness.

In the Hollywood blockbuster *Star Wars,* Obi-Wan Kenobi trains his protégé Luke Skywalker to become a Jedi Knight. Luke attempts to become proficient with his lightsaber but fails, despite his concentration and effort, because he doesn't connect with his inner self, his Instant Intuition. Then Obi-Wan blindfolds him and tells him, 'Follow your feelings, Luke! Feel the force!' As Luke lets go and trusts his inner voice, he masters the use of the lightsaber.

As you develop spiritually and become more aware of your own aura, you will become more confident with your psychic abilities and you will feel the force within you. You will also feel more open to other people's energy, and this will help you to deal with them and find out what they're really like as people. Here are a few of my favourite exercises which I teach my students and which will also help you to develop 'feeling' and 'seeing' energy.

Energy Ball

This exercise will help you to become aware of your own energy field. It is subtle, but once you get the hang of it you will become aware of your entire energy field and just what you can do with it.

1. Hold your hands out in front of you, palms facing each other and about 25 centimetres (10 inches) apart. Slowly move your palms towards each other. At some point you will feel a slight ball of energy almost like a bubble. Keep moving your hands, push them slowly towards each other but don't let them touch. Feel the energy and play with it. Feel your hands bounce on and off it. Cup your hands and feel the ball build up energy.

2. Now rub your hands together briskly for at least five seconds and again bounce your hands towards each other. The energy will be stronger now and you may well feel as if it is trying to push your hands apart. Move your hands backwards and forwards and feel the invisible sponge bouncing between your hands. This is your etheric energy.

No matter what your strengths, you will be able to feel energy. You have already been aware of it at times when you have 'felt' someone standing too close to you. Or when you have 'sensed' someone staring at you. Their energy field has touched yours. You have been aware of it when you have said, 'We're on the same wavelength.'

Types of psychic

There are different types of psychic, so it might be useful for you to find out at this stage of your development whether you're *clairsentient*, *clairaudient*, *clairvoyant* or an *empath*. Once you are aware of your energy fields and those of other people, you will instantly know whether you and that person 'connect'.

Clairsentients 'feel', so, if they're in an old building, they will pick up emotions and perhaps events that have happened possibly many years beforehand in that property or location. They will say things such as,

'The hairs on the back of my neck stood on end.'

'That gave me the willies.'

'There's something about him that gets under my skin.'

Clairsentients are often skilled at psychometry because they are in tune with feelings and so can pick up impressions left on objects.

Clairaudients 'hear', so, in the same situation, they might pick up voices or snatches of conversation. They are usually telepathic and can tune into people's thoughts and emotions. They say things such as,

'I feel in tune with you.'

'Something tells me this is odd.'

'A little voice is telling me not to go there.'

Clairaudients make good mediums and communicate well with spirits.

Clairvoyants are 'visual'. They usually see pictures in their mind's eye. Some can even visualise as if they were watching a mini-movie of events. They can be very influenced by their dreams. They say things such as,

'I don't like the look of this.'

'From what I can see this is wrong.'

'This place is rather dark.'

Clairvoyants – because of their visual skills – have an affinity with tarot cards.

Empaths literally do empathise with others. The word comes from the Greek *empatheia*, meaning 'passion', and *patheia*, meaning 'to experience suffering', and to an extent this is true. Many empaths will actually feel what others are feeling, even over long distances. This sensation can be emotional or physical. Most healers are empaths. They connect with the person they are healing and know where their problems lie without being told.

In fact, we are all empaths to an extent. At some point you have 'felt' that someone close to you was unhappy, in pain or troubled. When I went into labour with my first child, my life-long friend Leslie packed a bag and headed for her car, telling her husband, 'I'm off to Slough – Anne's gone into labour.' He told her not to be so daft because I wasn't due for several days, and besides, no-one had telephoned and most first babies are a few days late. Leslie drove from Northampton and arrived just before I gave birth. As you can imagine, I was very pleased to see her.

Many people have also told me stories of how they called their sister because they knew she was in pain, or their brother who was in trouble.

The key is to work with and use your strengths because they are your natural gifts. Many people try to be good at everything, but this can have the effect of watering down your abilities and making you a jack-of-all-trades. Once you feel confident with your main skill, you can work on others to give you a broader range, but I know many highly gifted psychics and healers who just use their main sense.

As I've said, and I'll say it again, all psychics work with energy. It's how we pick up information because we are simply more sensitive to it and are able to interpret it. Some psychics translate the information by way of pictures in their mind's eye, some simply 'feel' or just 'know'. Whatever method they use, they are still working with energy.

During one of my psychic-development workshops, which explores the concept of energy, I ask the group to focus on one person at a time and to feel the person's aura. They each write down what they pick up, which can be thoughts, images, a sensation or colours. The class are astonished to find that most of the participants 'see' the same things for each participant. Recently, I decided to have some fun. During a meditation I told the group to expand their auras to make them bigger and brighter. I watched the group and saw each and every one of them shine out. I jokingly said, 'The next time you want to get attention just do this, expand and brighten your aura. Do it at a party. You will definitely get noticed.'

That night one of the girls in the group, Cosima, went to a nightclub with her friends. She told them, 'Just watch me. I'm going to make my aura really bright, then everyone will notice me.' Her friends laughed and told her she had lost the plot. As Cosima walked across the room to the bar, every male head in the place turned to follow her. Cosima is a really pretty girl, so I am not that surprised. But she also told me, 'I've never known anything like this. The girls stood watching with their jaws dropping open. They said, "Whatever it is you're doing, teach us!" So I did.' So, if you can't take your eyes off someone in a bar, it might be because they've turned up their aura.

··

Turning up your aura

The first time you try this technique you will need to find a quiet place and relax. After a few practice runs, you will be able to do this anywhere and at any time.

1. Close your eyes and imagine your aura surrounding you. Just visualise feeling your aura and don't worry too much about actually seeing it. Simply build a picture in your mind's eye of it stretching out from your body.

2. Now see that the colours are made up of energy, which dances around you. Take your first impressions to find out your colours. Try it now. Immediately think of the first three colours that come into your mind. They may appear visually as colours, or as words, or you may 'hear' them. In whatever way you pick up this information, your Instant Intuition has just told you three of the colours in your aura.

3. Once you know the colours of your aura you can begin to visualise them around you. A great exercise is to sit quietly and imagine your aura. Be aware of how each colour feels. Next, imagine increasing the brightness of each colour to make your aura really shine and glisten. As the colours increase in intensity you will feel the characteristics of that colour flow through you. It feels marvellous.

4. Now experience the energy vibrating and shining and be aware that this energy is part of you and so it can be controlled by you.

....

Recently, I decided to try something out. I had been practising making my aura shine when I wanted to be noticed and also drawing it in when I wanted to be incognito. And there's one particular acquaintance who I definitely wanted to avoid. Whenever I was in town she would appear out of nowhere and talk for ages about nothing. She would tell me how she had washed her kitchen floor and peeled her potatoes. I'm a tolerant person but she drove me crazy and often made me late for appointments! One day I was walking to the local post office when I saw her on the other side of the road. This woman had eyesight an eagle would be proud of. She could spot someone from a mile away. I drew in my aura and dulled it down. I imagined it to be a smoky grey. She walked right past without noticing me. I realised that this could have been a fluke but I intended to practise.

During the next workshop I turned my aura, using visualisation, into a bright fountain coming out my crown chakra – the energy centre at the top of your head (see Chapter 4 for more on chakras). I actually wrote down on a piece of paper that my aura would be like a Roman candle spouting out of the top of my head. It was now my turn for the group to look at my aura. Two people wrote down, 'It looks like you have a bright golden light spouting out of the top of your head.' There were a few shocked faces when I showed them the piece of paper.

As you work with the exercises in this chapter you will begin to actually notice a slight glow around people, something like the halo you see around car headlights on a rainy day. Allow it to just happen naturally because if you try too hard it will be less likely to occur. Remember that this is a natural skill and it will happen best when you are relaxed. The 'Let's Sparkle' exercise that follows is a simple introduction to becoming aware of your own energy field.

....

Let's Sparkle

1. Sit in a quiet room with subtle lighting, and slowly move the fingers of each hand towards those of the other. Do this very slowly. If you watch and focus, you will see little sparks of energy flash off the ends of one set of fingers towards those on the other hand.

2. You can do this with a small pet. Hold your hands in its direction and imagine the sparks flying off the ends of your fingers and towards the pet. I do this with my cats. They always look around, often with that 'why are you bothering me?' look. Don't worry – it doesn't harm them at all.

This sparking energy is similar to the static you create when you brush your hair or when you rub a balloon on your jumper to make it stick to you.

....

The 'Green Fingers' exercise that follows helps you to get used to seeing different energy fields.

··

Green Fingers

You can do this exercise with any plant but I like tomato plants. You can buy a tomato plant or grow it from seed. Keep the tomato plant in a pot and each day look at it in subtle lighting similar to the light at dusk. Put the plant against a plain background. You may wish to experiment between a light and dark background – some people prefer light, some dark. Study the plant and allow your eyes to go slightly out of focus and look around the plant, not at it. You will begin to notice a glow of energy around the plant.

Each day as the plant grows you can notice the energy field. As the tomatoes arrive, watch them grow and notice how big their energy field is, even when the fruit is tiny. When the fruit is ripe enough to eat, remove it from the plant and each day study the energy field and notice how it gradually diminishes.

You can also study the energy field of sprouting foods such as alfalfa. Their etheric vibes are often huge because these tiny sprouts contain a huge amount of energy.

If you practise every day you will develop a keen etheric eye, which is handy for checking out how fresh your food is at the supermarket. Some people find it easier to see the energy field of plants and people if the room is dark and they place a torch behind the subject.

After practising seeing the etheric energy around plants and playing with energy, you will be ready to try to see the human aura. The aura around a plant is quite different from that of a human being or animal – often it's more dense and shinier but doesn't contain as many colours. By the way, if you don't physically see the energy field around a person you may well just 'see' it in your mind's eye or you may just 'know' what it looks like or even 'feel' it.

In one of my workshops a young man called Carl looked upset and said, 'I can't see anyone's aura. Everyone here seems to be so much better than me.' So I told the group to focus on one particular person and asked them to write down what they could see. I suggested to Carl, 'Write down what you *feel* the colours are in the person's aura.' Everyone except Carl 'saw' dark blue-green or a dark greeny blue. Carl was astonished to learn that he had 'felt' the same colours. His dominant psychic sense was obviously clairsentient (sensing) as opposed to clairvoyance (seeing).

The human aura is glorious and once you have the knack, just sitting outside a coffee shop sipping your latte and watching passers-by will be a joy. Here are a few exercises you can try to speed up your exciting new talent.

Seeing the Human Aura

1. Ask a friend to stand against a dark or light background (you may wish to try both). Soften the lights and relax and breathe deeply. Make sure that you are standing at least 1 metre (about 3 feet) away from them and ask them to stand still and allow their body to feel comfortable. This will work a lot better if they are not standing to attention!

2. Allow your eyes to go slightly out of focus and look through the subject and not at them. Close your eyes, feel their aura. What is its colour? Open your eyes and walk over to them

and gently hold your hands about 15 centimetres (6 inches) from their shoulders and tummy. What colours do you feel? You may have the same feeling now as you had when you held the ball of energy between your palms (see 'Energy Ball', page 73), after rubbing them.

3. Now stand a few feet further away and again allow your eyes to go slightly out of focus and look through your subject. Can you see a glow? It may look like the glow around a street lamp or candle. Are there any colours? Can you see the energy moving? What do you feel this tells you about your subject?

4. Ask your subject to sway their hands gently back and forth. This works best if there is a light behind them. Look out for a light trail behind them that looks a little like petrol fumes.

....

If you find you can clearly see or feel someone's aura, you may wish to study this further. By studying a person's aura you can pick up information about their physical, emotional and spiritual wellbeing. You can tell if there have been times of great upset and upheaval in their lives and you can work to strengthen their aura by studying aura soma and other forms of colour therapy.

You may instinctively know what colours the person needs because your instincts will act as a guide. You may think, 'This chap has so much red in his aura that it makes him hot-headed – he needs some ice blue to cool him down.' Or someone with lots of pastel colours may need a splash of something stronger to make him or her more dynamic. You can suggest that they imagine breathing in the colour or eat foods of the required shades. For example, if someone needs yellow, it usually means they're down in the dumps or a little 'grey'. They can eat bananas, yellow peppers and sweetcorn to bring sunshine energy into their body. They might also like to *wear* yellow – even if it's just a pair of socks hidden beneath their trousers.

The colour purple

Before we try another exercise, let's take a look at a very brief outline of aura colours and their meanings.

Red: High energy, confident and strong. Too much red can denote anger or indicate that you will burn out.

Pink: Loving and kind, usually a sign that you help others. Too much pink can mean you're a soft touch or live with your head in the clouds.

Orange: Creative and sociable. Too much orange can make you self-indulgent.

Yellow: Intelligent, logical and creative. Too much of this colour can make you overcritical or think too much, which can lead to your becoming bogged down in detail.

Green: Hardworking and reliable, you can be ambitious. Too much green can result in your not having enough fun.

Blue: Caring and loyal. You can be sensitive, but too much can isolate you.

Violet/purple: Unconventional, lateral thinker and spiritual. Too much can result in your living in a fantasy world.

White: Highly evolved, connected to the universal energy and aware of your soul purpose.

Gold: Very special and usually seen only in the auras of Spiritual Masters, shamans, gurus and other holy people.

Now you have the basics for feeling, sensing and seeing energy, including the aura, you're ready to move on to developing the Etheric Energy Technique. EET is actually an umbrella term I've devised to describe a series of techniques that use etheric energy to tap into people's emotions and create energy walls of protection around people and property. It can even influence another person's actions. Here, I'm just going to teach you how to tap into someone's thoughts. You will be able to use this skill at work and in your personal life. Before you do any psychic work, remember to protect yourself using the exercises outlined in Chapter 2.

Etheric Energy Technique

Have you ever been in a car with a satellite navigation system? The system is amazing – the box sits on your car's dashboard and actually speaks to you and guides you to a preprogrammed destination. 'Take the next left. Now go straight over the next roundabout,' it tells the driver. Just imagine having a little voice like that with you all the time, telling you which way to go in all areas of your life. 'Don't go to David's house tonight, he'll be in a bad mood. Go to Caroline's flat – she has a few friends coming over. It'll be a scream.'

If you get in touch with your Instant Intuition you will be able to tune into your own spiritual satellite navigation system. You have a little voice inside you waiting to guide you. You just need to learn how to listen. Last year a close friend, John, an IT manager, asked me to go with him to his boss's wedding. I agreed, but deep down I had an uneasy feeling. It was nothing dramatic – something just didn't feel right. The trouble was, the feeling wasn't overpowering and normally in these circum-stances most people tend not to take any notice.

I admit I fell into this trap. We all expect fireworks or something to fall from the sky as a warning, and just a simple 'feeling' isn't enough to make us stop and listen. But we need to recognise this feeling as a subtle warning. The good thing is that, once we recognise the sensation, we will instantly know it's a sign. It's a bit like those old weather forecasters years ago. There was one, a Yorkshireman called Bill Foggitt who every day told the country on live TV what the weather would be like for the next few days. He would say things like, 'If my big toe gives a twinge there'll be frost by morning.' He was invariably right.

But back to the wedding. The happy groom had quickly made my friend feel an integral part of the IT company. He had even given him an unexpected pay rise after three months to show his appreciation for all his hard work. But that morning I took forever to get ready, which is unlike me. On the way to the wedding my friend said to me, 'Take the next left.' I drove straight on, then turned right. I knew this was the wrong way but I felt compelled to do it. I have spoken to other people who have since had the same experience. They have told me, 'I really don't know why I went that way. Deep down I knew I was heading in the wrong direction.'

We arrived at the wedding and everyone was perfectly polite and friendly. But I still had an uneasy feeling, almost butterflies in my stomach, and I couldn't wait to leave. With all my experience, I really had no excuse for not listening to my instincts. But somehow I began beating myself up, thinking, 'Anne, you really need to relax. Why are you so suspicious of people? They're really sweet.' Two weeks later John's boss sacked him. It turned out that they were plotting against him. Obviously the wedding invitation was a sneaky way of putting him off the scent of betrayal.

We all have that psychic niggle. You have had niggles like this before and may have ignored them. Or did you listen? If I had stopped and listened to my niggle I would have used my EET and tapped into what was going on. I could have saved my friend a lot of stress and upset. By the way, later he managed to get a large golden handshake, thanks to my identifying the single person on the board of directors who felt he was being treated unfairly. How did I find out his friend among 12? I used EET and it's an easy technique to learn.

Just recently I was sitting drinking green tea in a place frequented by the rich and famous. At that moment a very well-known female singer walked through the door. I was curious about what was going on in her life because I had heard many rumours and so I used my etheric energy to tap into her. I immediately felt that she was worried and upset about her husband. The feeling was so strong I quickly pulled away. I then sent her healing and love. Just the tiniest connection will give you a wealth of information in the same way a tiny piece of a hologram will show you the whole picture.

EET – The Five-Step Process

While this is a safe technique, if you feel anything that makes you uncomfortable, pull back immediately. You only need a sliver of information to tap into because this works in an instant on a high vibrational level. By briefly connecting with the person *you* will feel what *they* are feeling.

Step 1. First, become aware of your aura and feel its energy. Imagine making it brighter or duller, as we learned earlier. Now imagine the white glow of the etheric energy surrounding your aura. Once you have an awareness of your etheric energy you can do amazing things with it.

Step 2. Imagine moving your etheric energy, stretching it. Hold out your arms in front of you and imagine the etheric energy stretching way beyond them, extending two, three and four metres out in front of you, out of your fingers. Now, bring the energy back into your body.

Step 3. Next, allow your etheric energy to make a pointy shape on the top of your head and make it point up like a dunce's hat. Then bring it back. Play around and try out some ideas of your own.

Step 4. This is the important part. Now that you have 'found' your etheric energy, focus on your solar-plexus area and imagine your etheric energy forming a shape a little like an arm, and allow this to stretch out in front of you. Imagine this has a hand on the end.

Step 5. Now think of someone you come across in your everyday life, maybe a colleague or friend, ideally someone whose feelings you would find it useful to know. Take the etheric 'arm' and place the 'hand' gently on their solar plexus. This area is the seat of all emotion and is where you will find out exactly what you need to know. Take your immediate impression, don't censor it.

When you do connect with someone, it is vital that you do so for honourable reasons only. I see no difference between, on the one hand, studying body language to read someone or learning neurolinguistic programming (NLP) to discover what they are really thinking and feeling and, on the other hand, using EET to gain the information you need. So if you are using this on the person interviewing you for a job, that is fine, but if you use it to manipulate someone or simply to be nosey, you will receive misinformation. The universe won't be impressed with you if you abuse such a skill!

Top tips for practising EET

◆ Wait until you have plenty of time and are not going to be disturbed. Unplug the telephone.

◆ It may help to have soft background music and the sweet smell of a scented candle.

◆ Dim the lights and let your conscious thoughts float away.

◆ The key is not to put yourself under pressure. If it happens, it happens. If not, then maybe you are not meant to experience it at this moment. As soon you try too hard, the link will break.

A few months ago I used this particular EET technique to find out why I was finding a certain lady so difficult to deal with in my work. She was awkward and argumentative. As soon as my etheric 'arm' touched her solar plexus, I immediately knew that she was afraid of losing her job and felt out of her depth. After this I knew exactly how to interact with her. I helped her and gave her reassurances and we ended up with a great working relationship.

However, as with any energy work, especially where you use visualisation, you need to ensure that you don't psychically bring anything back when you use EET. I cannot stress enough how important it is for you to make sure there is no continued psychic link. Below is a simple exercise which will ensure that you protect your own energy field.

Breaking the Link

Follow this two-step process for 'sealing off', or breaking the psychic link.

1. After finishing any work using EET, imagine a pure-white sword cutting any bonds between you and the person you have been tapping into. You may see the cords as a flash in your mind and they could appear as anything from a golden rope, or ropes, to tree branches. Some people see them as white wiggly pipes! However they appear, imagine the link being severed.

2. Then fill your solar plexus area with light and seal the cords of the other person with light and send them the thought 'love' along with the colour pink, which vibrates to the frequency of love.

Case study

My friend Lauren, a make-up artist, had been with her partner Joe, a teacher, for two years. But suddenly he became very aloof. He began spending more time away from her and spoke little when they were together. Lauren was beside herself. She loved him very much and only two months before they had talked about marriage. She repeatedly asked him what the problem was, but all he would say was that he was just tired. It was obviously something far more serious.

Usually Joe would stay at her place at least four nights a week but lately it was two nights or less. I decided to use my etheric energy to see just what was going on. I turned my etheric energy into a tentacle and concentrated on Lauren's partner. I immediately saw a vision of him sitting on his bed back at home. He looked forlorn. This immediately put Lauren's mind at rest because she was worried he had met someone else or was out partying every night.

As my etheric hand rested on his shoulder I could feel his feelings. I later told her, 'He's worried that you'll outgrow him because your career's taken off so quickly recently. His own career isn't very good and he's losing confidence. I can feel that a good holiday would put you two back on track. Somewhere that he's always wanted to go to. Would that be Mexico?'

Lauren looked at me in astonishment. 'How did you know that?'

I replied, 'When I use my etheric energy to tap into someone, I can ask questions and get answers. I simply asked where you should both go on holiday.'

Lauren said, 'Anne, that's incredible. You've always picked up on people for me before, but that's very precise.'

I suggested Lauren come along to my next class, so she could learn to use her own energy and immediately know what was going on with the people in her life.

Your etheric energy is very pliable. Just recently I had lunch with a top television presenter at a well-known TV studio. As I explained etheric energy to him he looked dubious, so I told him how to make the energy into a tentacle and reach out and touch people.

He followed my instructions and 'tapped' a nearby producer on the shoulder. He nearly jumped out of his skin when she suddenly looked around. They exchanged pleasantries, and then she smiled and said she had been meaning to set up a meeting with him because she had a project he might like to work on. He later said to me that he would definitely be using it in the future to gain someone's attention. When you're involved in an industry like the media, which relies on networking and contacts, it's a great tool to help you grab someone's attention in a crowded room or at a party.

Fine-tuning your EET

As I mentioned earlier, sitting outside a coffee shop watching the auras of passers-by is fascinating. You can do the same with EET. I like to sit in the coffee shop of a train station and watch people bustle by. Every so often, pick someone out and use EET to tap into them. What do you feel? Where are they heading? To work, on holiday, meeting a lover? Are they happy? Stressed?

Full of anticipation? By the time you have connected to a few dozen people you will have honed your skill and will be able to gain a quick snapshot of anyone in an instant.

Once you know how to tap into people you can do this over any distance. A client of mine, Mike, a top entrepreneur, was thinking of investing in a company overseas. The business partner was a chap he had known for years and who had been very successful. Mike came to see me because something was niggling him. He said, 'I just can't get a handle on it.' I taught him to use EET to tap into his prospective business partner. Mike jumped back into his seat and said, 'Crikey he's nearly bankrupt. No wonder he wants me involved – he needs my money to bail him out.'

Mike carried out some investigations and found the information to be true. He told me, 'In future I'll have a peep before I sign on the dotted line.'

This story may sound far-fetched but etheric energy can travel miles. Remember, everything is energy according to quantum psychics, and etheric energy is very real. Numerous scientific studies, including the work carried out by the Californian polygraph scientist Cleve Backster (see below), prove its existence, and some even show how we can send this energy out to people. This would explain why we know when someone is about to contact us – a little bit of their etheric energy 'taps' us on the shoulder.

The power of thought energy

Over 40 years ago Cleve Backster, a pioneer in polygraph (lie-detector) techniques, used a polygraph to detect whether a dracaena – a tropical evergreen plant – responded to a recent saturation watering with a change in the electrical resistance of its leaves. He subsequently discovered that the moment he *imagined* burning a plant leaf, the needle on the GSR reacted dramatically, indicating that the plant was distressed by what it perceived as a threat – Backster's thoughts.

Backster then devised various experiments in the field he now calls *biocommunication*. In his first published experiment, he demonstrated that monitored plants react to events such as tiny brine shrimp dying in boiling water in the lab. He then went on to take swabs of saliva from people and suspend these in a saline solution. The white cells in this solution were then monitored and found to react to the donor's emotions and actions even when they were miles away.

He took the white cell samples, then sent the people home to watch an emotional programme on television (such as a war movie), then videotaped both the programme and the response of the subject's cells. What he discovered was that cells outside the body still reacted to the emotions the person felt, even though they were maybe miles away.

Backster says, 'The greatest distance we've tested has been about 300 miles ... we find plants responding to our intentions, our thoughts, and we get plants reacting to the death of other creatures.'

Backster continues to pursue plant and cell-monitoring research as head of the Backster Research Foundation, as well as teaching in the Backster School of Lie Detection in San Diego. The implications of his work are staggering. It is scientific proof that our thoughts can be picked up as energy and affect living things around us, and it finally proves what spiritual teachers have been telling people for years. We are all interconnected. We are all one. Everything is energy, even thoughts. This is how telepathy works – by sending thoughts to another person you are sending them mental energy. I found this hard to understand at first until someone explained to me that it is no different from a radio sending out words and music over great distance. In effect, telepathy is energy floating from one place to another.

The psychic twins

Kelly and Stacey Franklin are identical twins – but are alike in more ways than meet the eye. They've shared a psychic link since childhood. They even claim they can communicate tele-pathically and are a fantastic example of how two people have developed and use their Instant Intuition instinctively.

Stacey says, 'As soon as we could talk we've been able to communicate telepathically. The messages don't come out as sentences – it's more a condensed thought with lots of meaning. I can look at my sister and know exactly what she's thinking and feeling, and she can do the same for me.

'Our psychic skills didn't go unnoticed. My parents have been aware of our link for a long time. My dad first started setting us ESP [extrasensory perception] tests when we were eight. He used to put me in the living room and Kelly in the kitchen and then ask us to draw the first picture that came into our heads. For ten minutes or so, we'd sit alone happily scribbling away. Then when we'd finished, we'd both show our dad.

'Often we drew dogs in parks, houses with ponds, big trees, the detail was always identical right down to the wacky colouring pencils we picked out to use. At first, Dad was convinced we were teasing him, that we'd worked it out beforehand, but we never did.'

Kelly adds, 'One time at school – we were about fifteen – our teachers were convinced we were cheating in our exams, so they put us in different rooms for a maths test. I think they were probably carrying out their own sort of experiment, like Dad. We both came out with the same mark, 91 per cent, by answering the same questions in exactly the same way.

'I remember our maths teacher being totally amazed, saying, "It's not possible" when he told us about it. But it was, and we'd sat in separate rooms. That's a good illustration of our telepathic link.

'Being twins we're used to finishing each other's sentences and knowing instinctively what each other is thinking, so we never talk over the top of each other. It might sound weird to some people but we've spent all of our lives together. From the minute we were born, we were in cots next to one another and as children if we were separated for more than a few minutes we'd start to look for one another. My sister is my best friend and she knows me better than anyone – which isn't surprising, considering she can read my mind.'

While you might not be able to communicate telepathically like the psychic twins, you can certainly use EET in all areas of your life to find the answers to life's important questions.

How to use EET in your own life

I've taught this technique to numerous clients and friends. Here are a few examples of how they have used EET to help them tackle important issues.

◆ A woman found the house of her dreams but when she tapped into the buyer she found he had no intention of selling at all. She didn't waste her time on an expensive survey.

◆ A friend needed to get her hair cut for an important job interview. Her own hairdresser was away, so we used EET to tap into a nearby stylist. We both agreed that he would rush her hair and make a mess of it, which would leave her feeling self-conscious during the interview. We found her an alternative salon which gave her a brilliant haircut! Since then, my friend has heard on the grapevine that the first stylist has got a bad reputation for rushing, especially on a Friday when he wants to go out with his friends for a drink.

◆ A client who runs a global business found the snake in the grass in his work situation. How? He tapped into his list of possible suspects and found the traitor.

Other possible areas to use EET
Use EET . . .

◆ before agreeing to go on a date

◆ to discover why someone is upset or moody

◆ to find out what someone's real intentions are in any given situation – personal or private

◆ to find a kindly dentist

◆ to decide which boss to work for or which project team to join.

One of my friends tapped into a cosmetic surgeon in Los Angeles. What she felt gave her doubts but because his credentials were so good she went ahead. He did an okay job but she didn't feel it was the best. Later, she heard he'd been struck off. EET has many varied uses – I've even tapped into a restaurant and found what I can only describe as a 'sneaky energy'. Some friends later ate at this place and suffered from terrible food poisoning.

Once, my partner and I were invited to stay with a couple who live overseas. It was a last-minute trip so we didn't use EET until we were on the plane. We felt great anxiety and stress around the couple and we arrived just as they were having a huge row. She had been seeing a married man across the road and her husband found out just at that moment. Luckily, there was a good hotel up the road. If I had tapped in earlier, I could have saved us an awkward situation. On the plus side, I've used EET to find everything from the right garage to repair my car and to find my ideal cat out of a litter.

So now you've learned how to sense and/or see energy and how to tap into people's emotions. This is an ongoing skill that will improve the more you use it. Practise the exercises you've learned so far as often as you can, and you will notice a rapid growth in your Instant Intuition along with your ability to master your control over your own etheric energy.

It's time now to look at another way of tapping into information in a manner that should get you into the swing of things – quite literally.

CHAPTER 4
The Power of the Pendulum

I was learning a lot about my intuition and how to tap into it to find out more. But my journey was by no means over. In fact, the more I learned about how to use my intuition, the more I wanted to find out, so I continued to meet up with Greta for coffee. I would plague her every few weeks with questions about developing my skills and finding out about my own destiny. I was hungry to learn and grow from her great wisdom. My questions are probably very similar to the ones you're asking yourself now too:

◆ What am I meant to be doing with my life?

◆ What spiritual lessons do I still need to learn?

◆ Why does life sometimes feel like a struggle?

When I posed these questions to Greta she would just tap her head and repeat her earlier advice. 'You already know all the answers – it's all in here.' She would then add I was exactly where I was meant to be 'right now – and you're doing exactly what you are meant to be doing.'

Greta was telling me to 'trust the process', which can be so hard. We push our way through life and it's completely alien to surrender to a higher force we might not even be sure, or believe, exists. Yet when I did my readings for clients, I trusted the process and I didn't question the pictures and words that flowed into my mind – and I never do now. So why couldn't I do this in my own life?

One day I asked Greta, 'Why is it when I need to know something for myself it sometimes feels as if there's a block?'

She told me, 'When you're with a client you let go but you try too hard for yourself. You need a tool, something that will bypass your conscious mind.'

My ears pricked up, 'Like what?' I asked.

'Like the pendulum,' she said, smiling.

As I mentioned earlier, when Greta first entered my life she was known for her love of the pendulum. I thought back to the many times I had seen her use it to make decisions and find answers – and on one occasion when we were invited to a posh dinner she even dowsed the food. Greta held her pendulum over her meal and, lost in concentration as she focused on one item of food at a time, tested it to see if it was suitable for her to eat. She held the pendulum over a pile of peas. It gently swung positively. She smiled and moved on to the carrots. They too got a thumbs-up. Then she held the pendulum over several new potatoes, but there was a definite negative swing. Greta looked up and said, 'No more potatoes for me today.' The entire table stopped and stared. Greta didn't care one jot what people thought about her. She was very careful to eat a balanced diet and her pendulum had given her so much information over the years it was like an old friend. She trusted it implicitly.

If you can master the pendulum, you will have access to instant answers to all manner of things, from locating a great holiday destination to finding a wonderful job. Your own gut instinct, the sense everyone possesses, will steer you in the right direction – but your pendulum will give you finely tuned answers to such an extent that not only will you know which vitamins to take, but you will also discover how many. At the same time, your dowsing will help you to build a stronger connection to your Higher Self, which is the part of you that knows everything. You will develop the habit of taking your pendulum everywhere with you – it will be like having your very own genie in a bottle.

How I discovered the pendulum

My first brush with the pendulum came when I was in India. I had been sitting eating my breakfast by the roadside kiosk with Vikram and I had said to him, 'I wish I had a button on my arm and all I had to do was press it and I would be psychic.'

He laughed and said, 'There will come a day when you will not need such a button. You will just know. But there is a way of quickly accessing the place of all knowledge.'

Excitedly I asked him, 'Where is that?'

He replied, as he finished the last of his chapati, 'Within you. Watch this.'

From around his neck Vikram took a pendant. It was a round, metal plumbing washer hanging on a long piece of string. He held it out in front of him. 'I shall ask if it will be sunny tomorrow,' he said, with a twinkle in his eye.

'Vikram, it's always sunny. We're in India,' I replied, sighing.

'I know, but we shall ask anyway.'

The pendant slowly began to turn anticlockwise, then it picked up speed until it was spinning very quickly in a huge arc. I wondered if he was a conjuror but he assured me he wasn't.

'So how does it move?' I asked.

He told me, 'There is a part of ourselves that makes it move. This is telling me it will not be sunny tomorrow.' I laughed and said, 'Well, that's wrong.'

He showed me how to make the pendant move clockwise for a 'yes' answer and anticlockwise for a 'no' answer by merely concentrating on a question mentally. Then on the pavement, he traced a circle in the dust with his finger and said, 'Let us ask what is important to you.' In the circle he drew symbols and told me the shapes stood for various elements of my life: family, friends, study, work, love and health.

'Here, try yourself, just hold it still,' he instructed.

I asked the pendulum out loud, 'Is my name Anne?' I held the cord and watched the pendant slowly begin to move in a tiny circle. I felt the coarseness of the cord against my palm. 'So what is it made of?' I said, expecting him to say some kind of rope.

'It is from a horse's tail,' he said, laughing.

Suddenly the pendant picked up speed. It began to move most definitely over one of the strange symbols. Faster and faster it swung in a bold circle. I asked Vikram what the sign in the dust meant. 'Spiritual development – and this is no surprise to me. So now you must keep the pendulum and practise asking it questions. It will serve you well.' I was honoured he had given me his pendulum. It felt as if someone had given me the key to a secret box.

That night I used the pendulum to find out answers to every-thing I could possibly think of in all areas of my life. I asked about family, friends, who would win the next general election.

It gave such definite answers that I couldn't wait to tell Vikram. Unfortunately, the next day there was a freak storm and I didn't want to leave the ashram, so I had to wait another day before I could see him again. When I did, the first thing he said to me was, 'I told you it wasn't going to be sunny.'

After years of practising with this amazing instant tool, I've come to realise that pendulums bypass the conscious mind and allow the user to access information quickly. Since Vikram introduced it to me, it's become one of my favourite quick methods of divination.

Types of pendulum

Dowsing tools come in all shapes, sizes and materials. You can buy clear quartz pendulums, rose quartz offerings, small and large wooden points and even metal tools. I use a different dowsing tool depending on what I'm searching for at that given moment. I've even known dowsers to use hollow ones and put a tiny amount of the substance they're looking for inside them, such as gold, and then the pendulum guides them to it. Uri Geller is probably one of the most famous dowsers, and has used his gift to detect precious metals and oil. But dowsing can be used for anything from finding lost objects to finding water and even missing people.

Which pendulum?

Most experienced dowsers prefer a natural substance such as wood, metal or a crystal such as quartz, because natural substances come from the earth and are therefore more in tune with the universe.

But I really think it's up to you to experiment and try out all different types. One of my workshop attendees loves using her garage key as a makeshift pendulum, another prefers her wedding ring on a piece of string. In my gran's day, either a wedding ring or a curtain ring would be attached to a chain. The main thing is that the pendulum needs to be symmetrical and able to swing freely.

Whatever material you opt for, it's important to make your pendulum really personal to you. Carry it with you, hold it often and make it part of you. After a while you will feel as if the pendulum is an extension of your arm and once you experience this, you will find using it will be as natural as brushing your teeth.

Even now when I use this method to help a client with a problem, or any of a host of other issues, I think back to how my mother used her homemade pendulum to predict the sex of babies, and I recall how Vikram traced patterns in the dust to create questions for his divining tool. Both of them were connected to their pendulums and trusted them. You can, too.

Programming your pendulum

Before you start practising, you need to programme your pendulum specifically to you. Here's how.

◆ Hold your pendulum cord or chain in your dominant hand between your index fingertip and your thumb. Hold your arm out in front of you so that the energy can flow down your arm and into your pendulum. If you are holding your arm upright, it's harder for the energy to flow.

◆ Allow the pendulum to hang still, then in your mind, tell it to swing clockwise to represent a 'yes' answer. Once the pendulum swings clockwise it has been programmed always to give a clockwise motion for a 'yes' or positive answer.

◆ Now ask the pendulum to swing in an anticlockwise direction for a 'no' answer. Again, as your pendulum swings this way it has now been programmed to give an anticlockwise motion for 'no' or a negative answer.

> *Before you use any new pendulum, and at regular intervals, you should cleanse and energise it. But we'll look at that in more detail in 'Cleansing and energising your pendulum' on p. 113.*

One of the best pendulums I have used I 'borrowed' from a builder who left it behind in my house after doing some work. It was his metal plumb bob. It was very heavy and the cord was an old piece of string. I found that it responded to my queries very definitely – better than Vikram's horse-hair version which had long been lost!

Water, water!

Sir William Barrett, professor of physics at the Royal College of Science in Dublin from 1873 to 1910, and Theodore Besterman, lecturer at the University of London School of Librarianship, carried out a number of studies in the 1920s for finding water using various methods, including dowsers, geologists and consultant engineers. Their results showed that the dowsers located twice as much water as the engineers, while the geologists found virtually none.

How to ask questions

In one of my Instant Intuition workshops a young woman called Millie asked her pendulum, 'Will I be happy?' The pendulum refused to move because the question was too vague. What does she mean by 'happy'? Perhaps she will be happy in love but not in her career. Or perhaps she will be happy some days and not others. You have to be specific.

I find the best questions are the ones where we weigh up options such as which job to take or which house is a better buy. By wording your questions carefully, more specifically, you will receive more accurate answers.

Questions, questions! What to ask your pendulum

You can write a list and dowse this for the best option. To use this method, hold your pendulum in one hand and rest a finger of the other hand on the list you have written. Work your way down the list, asking the pendulum to move indicating 'yes' or 'no', and see which option gives you the biggest swing.

Or you may simply ask whether something is good for you or not at this particular time in your life. Here are some examples of questions you might ask, but of course the potential is limitless.

◆ Which friend should I visit?

◆ Whom shall I date?

◆ What company would be the best to work for?

◆ What foods make me stronger?

◆ Which career would I be best suited to?

◆ Is the promotion right for me?

◆ Is there a better alternative around the corner? (You can relate this to various questions concerning love, work, buying a house – anything).

◆ Which restaurant is most suitable for my lunch appointment?

◆ Where is my ideal holiday destination for this year?

◆ Who is the perfect hairdresser, plastic surgeon, dentist for me?

◆ Which car is most suited to me?

◆ Who would be a good mechanic for my car?

◆ Which Bach flower remedy do I need?

◆ Which zodiac sign would make the ideal friends/colleague/lover for me?

◆ Which vitamins do I need? (You may then dowse to see how many per day and then how long you need to take them for.)

◆ Which time or date is the best time for travel, shopping, meeting friends?

You can also dowse a chart to find out which area of your life needs attention. Here, I've sketched a chart with sections for 'family', 'social', 'work', 'love', 'money', 'study', 'sixth sense' and 'health'. You can use this chart or make up one of your own. If you want to use this method, allow the pendulum to swing gently over the diagram then close your eyes and wait until you feel a definite movement. Open your eyes and see which area your pendulum swings towards. This will be the area of your life you are meant to be dealing with at this moment. Again, if you need guidance, you can then use the list method which I've just outlined. For example, if the pendulum swings towards health

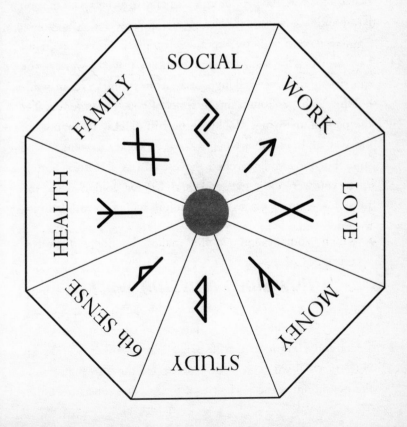

on the diagram, you could then write a list including such questions as 'Am I getting enough exercise?', 'Do I need to drink more water?' or 'Should I cut down on my alcohol consumption?'. By a process of elimination you will find your answer.

You can also dowse over a map. People often dowse over maps to find missing pets. Maybe you are trying to find a missing object, looking for relics or even the best spot to picnic. Simply hold your pendulum over the map. Now hold it over various spots for a few moments. You will find that over the areas which are not what you are looking for, the pendulum will either not move at all or it will move very little. Once you hit the areas that are for you, the pendulum will swing in a clockwise motion faster and faster.

If you need to look for something in a place where you do not have a map – for instance, your home or place of work – you can simply imagine walking slowly from room to room while holding your pendulum out in front of you. Observe whether the pendulum swings clockwise or anti-clockwise, or doesn't move at all. Remember when you were a child and someone hid something? As you searched they would say 'Hotter, hotter' when you were close to it and then 'Colder, colder' when you were in the wrong place. The pendulum will guide you in much the same way.

How does dowsing work?

By now you should asking, 'How does dowsing work?' As Greta and Vikram both told me, all the answers are already within us. All we need to do is to access the information and the pendulum is the perfect tool to link our conscious minds with our subconscious minds and, in turn, with the collective unconsciousness.

Collective unconscious is a term coined by the Swiss psychiatrist Carl Jung to describe that rich reservoir of shared instinct common to all human beings. In this realm – sometimes called the *superconscious* – are to be found what are known as *archetypes*, or universal symbols such as we meet in dreams and myth. These archetypes are common to all humans, irrespective of culture or ethnicity. You can see why your *superconscious* might be a fertile source of ideas and insights as you use your Instant Intuition to ask those important questions.

Have no doubt that we already know things before they happen, and you can tap into this information using your pendulum. The curious thing is, if you ask people if they ever have premonitions, they will tell you they don't, yet a number of laboratory tests conducted by Dr Dean Radin at the University of Nevada, Las Vegas, prove the very opposite to be conclusively the case. We do, in fact, know things before they happen.

Radin and his colleagues showed their subjects a series of slides. Most were of a peaceful nature, such as a landscape or someone smiling, but every so often they would be shown a slide of an autopsy or a pornographic image. The subject had two fingers on their left hand wired so that electrodermal activity (electrical activity in the skin) could be monitored. The slides were randomly chosen by a computer, ruling out any emotion or information that could have been unconsciously relayed to the subject by the researchers.

As you would imagine, when peaceful images flashed across the screen the subject was relaxed, and when the more extreme images were shown there was an increase in electrodermal activity. Now comes the interesting part. The electrodermal activity increased three to four seconds *before* the upsetting images appeared. Somehow the subjects knew a distressing image was about to appear on the screen. Yet later, when they were asked if they knew what picture was about to be shown, they said that they didn't have a clue. Somehow their subconscious mind could sense the images. Your pendulum will also enable you to bring this ability and information to the surface, because at this subconscious level you are tapping into that universal unconscious – Jung's *collective unconscious*.

What makes the pendulum move?

Hypnotherapists use what is known as the 'ideo motor response'. While their subject is in a trance-like state, they instruct them to allow one index finger to be the 'yes' finger and the other index finger to be the 'no' finger. They then ask their subject questions and allow the fingers to give the yes/no response.

A session would go something like this, 'Your left index finger is your "yes" finger and your right index finger is your "no" finger. When I ask you a question you may raise the appropriate finger in response.' The practitioner would then give their subject a simple question. For example, to a woman they may ask, 'Is your name Fred?' and their right index finger would then gradually rise upwards. They would then ask, 'Are you female?' The left index finger would then rise. Subjects are usually totally unaware of the movement because their answers are coming straight from their unconscious mind (the part of the mind that controls things that we do without thinking). For instance, when you walk to the shops you don't think through every step or say to yourself, 'Right, I'm going to turn now and step off the kerb'. Your movements are all done unconsciously. In hypnotherapy the subject's unconscious mind instructs their finger to move, even though they may not be totally aware that it is happening.

Going underground

Dr Zaboj Harvalik, a now-deceased Czech-American physicist, who for 25 years was professor of physics at Arkansas University, concluded from his research that dowsers are especially sensitive to electromagnetic radiation. They can also sense magnetic-field gradients from many things, including underground tunnels, pipes and moving water. He also conducted some ground-breaking studies in which he took dowsers and covered areas of their bodies with a metal shield. Harvalik found that certain areas acted like receptors or sensors. He pinpointed these sensors just below the solar plexus, slightly below the brain and in the area of the sinus complex.

Case study

Landscape gardener Rob doesn't need to rely on machinery to find underground pipes and cables. Instead he uses the ancient skill of dowsing. Standing in the large garden, he knows that underneath this pristine lawn there's a warren of pipes. One false move with his shovel, or mini-digger, and he could hit a pipe and cause mayhem.

'Hitting a mains is still an awful lot of hassle,' he says. 'When this happens you have to call out the utility services who usually turn everything off, which is such a pain for everyone.'

The normal way to avoid this problem is to use specialist electronic equipment. This sensitive machinery can pick up the location of the pipes, cables and suchlike, but hiring it can be expensive.

'However, I don't rely on modern methods,' says Rob. 'Instead, I use my dowsing rods. My Uncle Ken, a builder, taught me how to use the rods so it's a family skill. My uncle was always getting his rods out to have a look and see what was where, so he didn't hit a pipe in the floorboards.'

With practice, Rob became proficient and now has no qualms about using his divining tools. He explains, 'The rods are metal wires, which you can make out of old coat hangers, and you hold them gently in your hands and in front of you. You must tell them what you want to find and then when they hit that object, they cross.

'I always walk slowly around the garden or site I'm working on and draw a map of danger points to be avoided, or where I'm to dig gingerly. I've had a few raised eyebrows from clients, but most people are interested.

'You can feel the rods pulling with their own energy force. It's quite strange but you get used to it.'

Cleansing and energising your pendulum

The final area I wish to cover before you dash off and start practising with your pendulum is cleansing and energising it. You should cleanse your pendulum often. You do this by soaking it overnight in pure springwater with added sea salt. I really want to emphasise this ritual: it's very important if you intend to use dowsing for emotional or healing purposes.

If you are working on a health problem, or using pendulums often, you may need several. If so, you should rotate them to avoid them becoming overcharged with the negative energy that will have accumulated during the work the pendulum has done before.

Once your pendulum is cleansed, to energise it leave it lying on a window ledge on a sunny day and overnight when there is a full moon. The sun will give energy and the full moon will connect your pendulum to the universal force.

Once you are confident in your choice of pendulum, and it's cleansed and energised, you're ready to practise and explore your new spiritual skill. Like Greta, I now use the tool to dowse for everything from picking out fresh food at the supermarket to choosing a location for lunch. Yes, I use the pendulum if I need quick guidance to find out which restaurant has the right ambience for a particular meeting – be it with TV producers, for client consultations or a working lunch with a Hollywood scriptwriter. I write a list of the possible places, then I hold my pendulum in one hand and put my finger on each name, slowly keeping it moving down the list. When the pendulum swings in the direction for 'yes', I know I have the best meeting spot.

There are so many uses for your pendulum. This fantastic tool can give guidance on relationships, friendships, work and health – in fact, all areas of your life. The chart on page 107 will give you an excellent starting point but once you have used this diagram, you will be able to devise your own to help you decide anything you need to know at any given moment. I've outlined here the most important topics which I feel will make a major impact on your life.

The first exercise I ask my students to do at home on their own with their new pendulum is to check that they are sleeping in the right position in their bedroom, or that they are using the best room for their energy. One of the most important factors that can help you cope with the daily stresses of modern life is sleep. During sleep the body renews itself and the mind sorts out the day's events. The results of changing the position of your bed can be startling.

....

And So to Bed

To find out if you are sleeping in the right place, hold your pendulum over your bed and allow it to settle. Wait for a moment, then in your mind ask, 'Is this a good position for my bed?'

If your pendulum swings gently clockwise, then this is a good spot for you. If it swings wildly then this spot could give you a restless night. This can happen if you watch a lot of television in bed or have too many things around you, such as radios, CD players and even stimulating information, like magazines and books.

If the pendulum swings in a negative direction, this is not the spot for you, and if it stands still, this area has stagnant energy.

Have a clear-out, maybe paint the room a different colour, open the windows to let the air circulate and place a pure, clear-quartz crystal in that spot. The energy will soon clear.

If the energy is stagnant or negative, I would strongly suggest trying different positions in the room for your bed. You don't need to drag your bed around – simply place your pillow on the floor in different parts of the room. Note which spot gives you a gentle but definite positive spin. This will be the position in which you will need to point your feet.

....

Dowsing the chakras

We briefly met the chakras earlier, and I said we would come back to them. The word *chakra* comes from the Sanskrit meaning wheel or circle. Chakras are thought to be centres of psychic or metaphysical energy located at seven points in the body. The base chakra, represented by the colour red, is at the base of the spine. The sacral chakra is a little further up, in the pelvic region, and is represented by orange. Then there's the abdominal chakra, which is yellow or gold – by now you are probably recognising the order of the colours of the light spectrum. The heart chakra is next and is associated with green. The throat chakra is blue, and finally the head chakra is indigo and the crown chakra violet/white.

Chakras can be seen as spinning like a wheel, and by dowsing with your pendulum you can find out which chakras are spinning nicely and which are sluggish. By dowsing the chakras you can gain a wealth of information, because each one corresponds to a colour (as we've seen) and to particular areas of the body and emotions. If you find that a chakra is sluggish you can correct that area with your pendulum by eating foods of the colour associated with that chakra – adding to the missing energy. You can also bring the colours you need into your body by breathing them in – and I give a brief explanantion of this below:

Find yourself a quiet comfortable place to sit. Close your eyes and allow your whole body to relax. Concentrate on your breathing and allow it to flow naturally.

Now think of the colour you need and imagine breathing it in. For example, if you're low, imagine breathing in yellow. Just see it in your mind's eye as a yellow mist. Imagine it flowing to every part of your body right down to your toes, and flowing up to the top of your head. Even imagine it flowing to every cell of your body. Now imagine it flowing particularly strongly to its corresponding chakra point. See your chakra spinning healthily. As your chakra spins and glows with the colour yellow feel yourself energised and glowing with happiness because yellow is the colour of joy.

I am now going to give you two exercises to do as an introduction to working with your chakras. The first you can do either by yourself or with another person; the second will definitely require a willing friend.

....

A Chakras DIY

You can either use this method on another person or use your intuitive skills to dowse for yourself. Place one finger on the crown chakra on the diagram (page 118) and hold your pendulum in your other hand. Which way does it spin?

Clockwise shows a healthy energy flow, anticlockwise indicates an imbalance. Work your way down each chakra (very much in the way that I dowse for my lunching locations).

By using this method you can gain an instant result to find out if any of your chakras are out of balance and make the necessary adjustments, as discussed earlier, to regain equilibrium. When you're really practised, you won't even need a visual prompt and can just hold the pendulum in your hand and visualise each chakra point in your mind's eye. The pendulum will give you an instant result.

Practise on a friend

Now an exercise that you can do with a willing subject.

Make sure the room you are using is peaceful, dimly lit and sweet-smelling and perhaps play some soft music. Ask your subject to lie flat and make sure they are comfy. Explain what you're doing as you go along but make sure you speak in a soft and relaxed voice.

Hold your pendulum over each chakra beginning at the base. Focus your entire mind on just that one energy point. If you get a positive and definite swing you know that chakra is working well. Move on to the next energy point and so on.

The diagram on the next page illustrates where the chakras are located, which areas of the body they relate to, the colour associated with each one and the food to eat if it's out of balance – the colour going into your body will help to restore the energetic flow.

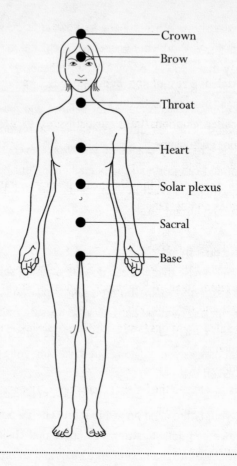

Crown

Brow

Throat

Heart

Solar plexus

Sacral

Base

The chakras

The base chakra

The base chakra relates to how grounded we are and balanced.

Associated areas of the body: spine, kidneys, bones, legs, feet

Associated emotions/traits: survival, strength, family and tribal connections, fears, anger

Colour: red

Foods to redress the balance: red apples, beetroot, cherries, radishes and strawberries

The sacral chakra

The sacral chakra represents our sexuality.

Associated areas of the body: gonads, reproductive system, adrenals, bowels and bladder

Associated emotions/traits: sexual issues, excitement, control, passion, guilt, blame

Colour: orange

Foods to redress the balance: apricots, oranges, carrots, mangoes and nectarines

The solar-plexus chakra

The solar-plexus chakra represents the seat of our emotions.

Associated areas of the body: pancreas, stomach, liver, gall bladder and nervous system

Associated emotions/traits: joy, responsibility, empathy, worry, confidence

Colour: yellow

Foods to redress the balance: bananas, coffee, eggs, grapefruit, lemons and olive oil

The heart chakra

The heart chakra, as its name suggests, is the energy point that relates to love.

Associated areas of the body: thymus, heart, blood, circulation, chest and lungs

Associated emotions/traits: love, happiness, balance, desires, hatred, loneliness, sadness

Colour: green

Foods to redress the balance: avocado, beans, cucumber, lettuce and spinach

The throat chakra

The throat chakra is related to how we express ourselves.

Associated areas of the body: thyroid, metabolism, alimentary canal, speech, tonsils

Associated emotions/traits: communication, truth, willpower, peace, tolerance, lies, addictions, criticism

Colour: blue

Foods to redress the balance: plums, grapes, blueberries

The brow chakra

The brow chakra deals with our intuition, study and thinking.

Associated areas of the body: pituitary gland, ears, eyes, brain, senses, nervous system

Associated emotions/traits: wisdom, self-knowing, understanding, accepting, fantasist, reckless

Colour: indigo

Foods to redress the balance: grapes, aubergines, blackberries

The crown chakra

The crown chakra connects us to the universe and our higher selves. It brings wisdom.

Associated areas of the body: pineal gland, brain, eyes

Associated emotions/traits: unconditional love, awareness, empathy, selfless, impractical

Colour: violet/white

Foods to redress the balance: rice, white fish, coconut

Dowsing relationships

As you can imagine, relationship issues are one of the many areas people come to see me about, and over the years I've been consulted by hundreds of people seeking guidance in this sphere of their lives. No doubt at some point you yourself will have looked at the person you're dating or living with and wondered, 'Is this the one?' You could be compatible with someone by talking to them for hours on end and having lots in common with them. You may fancy the socks off a person and spend many passionate moments. But the truth is that there is more than one way to be compatible, and this is one of the hardest of life's important questions to answer. Luckily for you, I've devised a quick test to give you some idea of your romantic success with any chosen person. It works on the law of compatibility. In any relationship there are four levels:

◆ physical

◆ mental

◆ emotional

◆ spiritual

Many couples who are very happy are compatible on just two levels. There is the odd rare pair who connect on all four but by dowsing you can see where you are compatible and where you are not. You can begin to decide whether this person is right for you. You can also simply identify areas that need working on to improve your relationship. Begin by taking a number of famous couples and assessing them using the charts that follow. Then write down your findings. It will be interesting at a later date to see how the celeb couple are getting along and how well you assessed them.

Often in my workshops we take couples in the limelight and each of us assesses their relationships. This helps to introduce people to the technique and the results can be quite fascinating. Many years ago we looked at Prince Charles and Princess Diana – they fell down on every level. If only they had consulted the pendulum first! We also looked at Prince Andrew and Sarah Ferguson when they got engaged. It showed that they matched very well emotionally but nowhere else. More recent examples include Hugh Grant and Jemima Khan Goldsmith, Brad Pitt and Jennifer Aniston, Jennifer Aniston and Vince Vaughn, Liz Hurley and Arun Nayar.

We've even checked out couples from history like Napoleon Bonaparte and his wife Josephine, Elizabeth I and her suspected lover Robert Dudley, and Cleopatra and Mark Antony!

....

True Love

Choose five famous couples from the present or from the past. Focus on one at a time and picture them in your mind. Now gently hold your pendulum in one hand and work your way down the list of the four levels below. Write down your findings and anything else you feel or information that comes to you. Using the pendulum can often quickly open our psychic minds.

Notice how firmly the pendulum swings to get an idea of just how compatible the couple are on each level. A big strong swing on 'emotional' could make up for quite a weak or negative swing on 'spiritual'. If you get a positive reading on any of the areas, this is what it means.

Physical: They will have a strong sexual and passionate relationship.

Mental: They are on the same intellectual level. They make a great partnership and will have plenty to talk about to stimulate one another mentally.

Emotional: They will have great empathy and understanding.

Spiritual: They are on the same path and have probably had past lives together. A wonderful connection.

The score

One out of four is **weak**.

Two out of four is **good**.

Three out of four is **wonderful**.

Four out of four is **hard to find**, so don't let this one go!

Make a note of your findings in your spiritual journal, as it will be interesting at a later date to see how the celebrity couple are getting along and how well you assessed them. Once you feel confident having practised with well-known faces, you are ready to try out this method in your own life. You can just focus on the four levels but other important questions concerning love could be, 'Can I trust this person with money?' or perhaps, 'Will they be faithful to me?' Or there may be a situation where you want to know if your partner is telling you the truth. Finding the answers to questions of the heart has to be one of life's biggest struggles, but it can be done easily and instantly.

To show you how using a pendulum for love works, I want to tell you the story about Geoff. He had been in a relationship for eight years and called it 'the longest engagement on record'. He and his girlfriend Charlotte were well suited and they did most things together. Yet after all this time neither had mentioned marriage, children or even moving in together. Geoff said, 'We really like each other. Charlotte is my best friend as well as my girlfriend. But it's as if we can't be bothered to take things further.'

The pendulum clearly showed they were very emotionally and mentally compatible, but the pendulum hardly moved physically or spiritually. Geoff said, 'You know, we rarely have a sexual relationship these days. I've often wondered what would happen if one of us met someone we really fancied.' A short time later, Charlotte met a man at work and married him within three months. Geoff admits he felt an element of relief and is now dating a gorgeous French girl, who he says has added 'a new spark to my life'.

Another one of my clients, Edwina, had been seeing Mike for six months. She adored him but had the feeling he didn't feel quite the same way about her. Yet he always told her he was crazy about her and often took her away and, as she put it, 'We have great sex all weekend.' Edwina found the only swing she got was on the physical. Emotionally, mentally and spiritually the pendulum hardly moved. Edwina said, 'I had suspected that Mike was a bit of a charmer and I worried that the relationship was little more than bonking.' Edwina confronted him and he admitted he had no intention of getting any more serious than the odd passionate weekend. The young woman decided to move on and meet someone new who she could have a deeper and more equal relationship with on more than just a sexual level.

Remember, relationships don't have to be purely of a sexual nature. We have relationships with friends, people at work, family members and our neighbours. If you want to find out how compatible you are with people in your sphere, you can (yes, you've guessed it) consult your pendulum. It can be interesting to keep a spiritual diary and make a note of how the scores go up and down over periods of time.

Match made in heaven?

Try the compatibility test on people in your life such as your best friend or work colleagues. This quick exercise can uncover all sorts of interesting developments. One of my students, Angie, found a big swing on the physical when she looked at her female boss. It turned out they made very good jogging partners.

Love dilemmas

If you want to know about a person you are dating, or are interested in, there are two ways to find out all you need to know about the situation. The first is to hold your pendulum over their photograph and focus on a question. Make sure the questions are framed very clearly – for instance, 'Does [name] care about me? Are we well suited? Would they make a better friend than a partner? Are they genuine?'

You can even dowse to see how long you will be together. You simply ask, 'Will we be together one year? Two years? For ever?' If the pendulum swings negatively on 'one year', ask whether you will be together one month? Two months? Work your way through the years. Remember, a negative swing concerning love doesn't mean you won't be together: it means a 'no' to that particular question.

The second method is to hold your pendulum, close your eyes and picture the person in your mind. Make sure the image of them is clear and vivid. As you imagine them, see them walking and smiling and even hear their voice. This will all help you to build a big connection. Now ask your pendulum your question.

At times, clients want to know whether their partner is having an affair. I ask them to write a list of possible names of the other party. Then at the bottom of the list I ask them to put a question mark. This represents someone my client hasn't met or simply doesn't know of. Below the question mark I ask them to put an exclamation mark. This represents someone the client would never suspect.

This technique proved very useful for my client Carole. She suspected her husband was seeing someone, and told me, 'It's probably someone at his work.' We dowsed together, each with a pendulum, and there appeared to be no hanky-panky around his job. We went through everyone she could think of, including women at his local pub. We then used the question mark. Again, nothing gave a positive swing. Next, we tried the exclamation mark, and both our pendulums swung wildly.

My Instant Intuition kicked in and I asked her, 'Is he involved in sport?' She told me he coached the local football team. I then asked, 'Is there a woman involved with this club?' Carole burst out laughing and said, 'She's so big she can hardly walk. Never!' I told her I truly suspected that this was the woman her husband was seeing behind her back. Carole is a tiny, good-looking woman and assumed her husband would be seeing someone younger and prettier, but, as is often the case, this was not so. She confronted him that evening and he confessed that he had been seeing the large lady for some time.

During my workshops, my students ask a variety of questions. There was Colin, for instance, who wondered whether his girl-friend would make a good mother. They had been together two years and he was very much in love with her, but she liked to party and he liked to stay at home. He wanted to ask her to marry him but was worried she would not settle down. We carefully asked a series of questions and discovered that she would still need a social life, but would be happy going out about once a fortnight. He left smiling and ready to propose.

Another client, Julie, wanted to know whether her boyfriend would stop spending so much money. For some time he had been asking her to buy a house with him but Julie had a few misgivings. She already owned a property, so she would have to sell up and put her capital into a new home. John was often short of money, at times borrowing from her at the end of the month. She didn't want to end up carrying a new and bigger mortgage on her own. We asked the pendulum if he would still overspend. The pendulum said yes.

Next, we wanted to find out whether he would improve with time. The pendulum slowly moved in a positive circle, showing yes. But because it moved slowly we gained the impression that it would take him a long time to learn not to waste money. I asked if John would improve his money-management skills if he had some session with a life coach. The pendulum gave a small yes.

Julie decided to ask him to move into her small flat for six months to see how things went. She could see there was a chance that he would become more responsible, but she wanted to see just how much before she committed. In the end, he did slowly grasp how not to let money slip through his fingers, and they later bought a house together.

Sally came to me because she wanted to know when her boyfriend would propose. We dowsed through the months and when we got to May the pendulum gave a definite swing. Sally shrieked and said, 'That's when he wants us to go on a holiday to the Caribbean.' She was adamant we hadn't spoiled her surprise. The next time I saw her, Sally was wearing a huge grin and a rather large diamond ring.

Dowsing for health

Another major use for dowsing is to do with health and healing. I have met doctors who, off the record, have told me they have dowsed to diagnose their patients' health problems, especially when they have been stumped for an answer. Few medical professionals would discuss this publicly. One, Dr S, told me, 'Although many people are open-minded these days, official bodies are not. You never know what the repercussions would be professionally.'

Dr S went on to tell me how he had a patient with a mysterious illness. He had sent her for every test he could think of and nothing had given even the slightest hint of the problem. 'I drew an outline of her on a sheet of paper,' he said, 'then gradually held my pendulum over each area until the pendulum gave an erratic response over the area of her pituitary gland. It changed direction many times and wouldn't settle into a clockwise or anti-clockwise spin, indicating a problem. I then dowsed through every conceivable problem to do with this gland until I found the malfunction. It was an obscure and little-known condition, but luckily cured in no time. My patient was better within days. I could tell you dozens of similar stories.'

He revealed that he had learned the technique while at a medical conference in France. He was astonished to find that many of the French doctors attending saw dowsing as a regular part of their work. One had taught him the technique during lunch and he had used it ever since to great effect.

Dowsing for your ideal diet

There are two ways of using this method. The first is to write a list of foods and dowse over each item to see which ones give you a positive or negative reading. Be sure to write the result beside each item in case you forget later. (We tend to have selective memory when it comes to things like chocolate!)

Also make a note of the strength of the swing – whether a wide or small circle. You will discover the foods that are particularly good for you and those that are definite no-nos. If your pendulum becomes very erratic, it is telling you that this reaction is what this food will do to you – it will make your body erratic. I usually find this points to an allergic reaction. Recently I dowsed a client and, when we came to cheese, the pendulum swayed wildly from side to side. She told me that cheese gave her severe migraines.

The second method is to hold your pendulum in your dominant hand and in your other hand hold an item of food. This gives you a very direct reading. You can use this method with another person by asking them to take an item of food and hold it while you hold their other arm and dowse. Again, some people may pooh-pooh this idea of testing food, but, as I always say, 'Make up your own mind and go on your own results.'

Consult your GP

You do not need me to tell you that if you have any concerns about your health you should consult your doctor. I know many people talk about alternative medicine, but I prefer to say *complementary*. We can all work hand in hand and conventional medicine has its place. I once had a major operation on my abdomen and without this conventional medical intervention I have no doubt I would have died.

Case study

Jim, a record producer, had felt out of sorts for some time when he came to see me. His energy was low, he was constantly tired and he had put on weight. His skin was also dull and spotty. As I dowsed first to check his body, I could tell his digestion was sluggish, leading to a build-up of toxins. Because I had visited him, I was able to test him against all the food in his fridge and pantry. The pendulum soon showed that he had a bad reaction to wheat and, much to his annoyance, the six-pack of lager in his fridge had to go. But, by radically altering his diet and his drinking habits, he was able to gradually restore his energy and health.

Case study

Julie, an experienced dowser, once told me, 'I pick up as much information from my body as I do with my pendulum. I receive different feelings for different answers. For instance, if I'm dowsing to see what the weather will be like, my knee will twinge if it's going to be cold or rainy that day – or on the date in question. My knee twinges slightly anyway, but it becomes so much more pronounced when I dowse. The pendulum alerts me so much sooner. It's as if the pendulum amplifies my senses.'

Dowsing for treasure

Another one of my friends, Bill, spends his weekends on Hastings beach and the nearby fields with his metal detector. He calls this his 'lucrative hobby'. Before he discovered dowsing, Bill would have good days and poor days detecting. Mostly he found coins dropped by holidaymakers but at times he came across a real treasure. Once he found a gold watch, which he handed in to the police. He has also found some ancient coins and an axe head.

One day a group of dowsers arrived at a field outside Hastings, where Bill was detecting. It was a cold, bleak day and Bill wasn't finding much and felt a bit dejected. The dowsers were great fun. They laughed and shared their warm soup with him. They also taught him to dowse. Bill told me, 'I had a wonderful day and now I also dowse to find the best spot to use my metal detector. My findings have trebled. Last week I unearthed several very rare coins. Dowsing has made this much more fun and I find a tidy sum now.'

Dowsing can be used to find any type of item, including leaks, which is especially helpful during a drought. Even UK water companies now admit to using dowsers. Southern Water in the southeast of England, which has a network of 13,500 kilometres of pipes, is on the record in the British media as saying, 'Fixing leaks is our top priority. We need to make sure we are doing everything we can to beat the drought. Divining is one of the techniques used by some of our crews, although by far the majority of teams use modern electrical equipment to measure flows and listen for noises of potential leaks and burst water mains.'

Dowsing can uncover many things, as we have seen in this chapter. But what about uncovering the past – not just the span of your current life so far, but a past going back centuries, or even millennia? This is something we'll look at next.

CHAPTER 5
How to Discover Your Past and Future

I will be forever grateful to Vikram for introducing me to the fantastic and ancient skill of dowsing and to Greta for fine-tuning my skills. I always thought Greta would be around for ever – you do, don't you? But then I had an unexpected bombshell. I came home and there was a message on my answerphone from Greta – she was disappearing to a retreat in Australia for three months and also planned to catch up with her son, who lived in this part of the world. Her last words for me were, 'You'll be fine, don't worry. Everything will work out just as it's meant to.'

When I heard the message I felt uneasy but I put it down to the fact that I was going to miss her stability, wisdom and guidance. While she was on the other side of the world, I heard very little about her whereabouts. The next piece of news was a phone call from Greta's husband Brian. I could hear the emotion in his voice as he told me, 'Greta's very ill. Can you feel anything Anne?' Hearing that my mentor and one of my closest friends was sick made the feeling of dread and panic well up inside, but this time it was almost overpowering. I took a deep breath to calm myself and replied, 'I feel she's hanging on by a thread but it'll be her decision to stay or go.'

Brian said, 'I feel much the same.'

The people that Greta had taught her unique brand of psychic skills to began communicating and the grapevine passed on the news. Greta's good friend Shelley, an astrologer, looked at her chart and told me, 'If she can hang on until Thursday she'll fully recover.' Greta passed away the day before this deadline. She was in her early 60s. I never found out exactly what she died from, it's not what you ask a grieving husband.

I was devastated and I was angry that my mentor had died. Why would someone who was such a shining light be taken suddenly? I felt lost and abandoned. I simply didn't understand why she had gone.

At her funeral, her friends, her colleagues and her husband Brian wanted to celebrate her life, but I couldn't go to the wake. I left after the service and I went home and sobbed on my bed. Deep down I knew Greta didn't want me to weep, so as a promise to her, I vowed to pass on her teachings and to help people from all sections of society. This is why you are reading this book now.

The vow acted as a catalyst because I went on to develop those revolutionary new techniques I've called EET, which have changed not only my life but that of everyone who's used them. Greta would have been proud of me.

Vikram taught me something else too, while I was in India in the 1970s. It was through him that I became interested in the concepts of reincarnation and karma, something I've been fascinated with ever since. Over 30 years ago, such ideas were virtually unheard of in Britain, but Vikram was adamant that I had experienced a previous incarnation in India. He told me,

'This is why you have been drawn to this country. It is your spiritual home. You have unfinished business here.' I asked him what the unfinished business was and he replied, 'That is for you to discover.'

During our chats by the Howrah Bridge, which stretches over the River Hooghly, Vikram told me about his many incarnations. As people passed by with bundles on their heads, he revealed the past life that had the biggest impact on him. It was his previous incarnation as a wealthy businessman. 'During this existence I lost sight of what is truly important in life. I lost my way on my spiritual path,' he said. 'I decided to come back this time as a beggar to teach myself to be humble.'

My instant reaction was, 'You *decided*?'

Vikram answered, smiling, 'Indeed. In between lives we decide many things – what role we will play, who we will meet in our lives and what we will learn. You have people in your life now that you have known in a previous existence.'

My mind boggled at this concept. 'Who?' I asked.

He replied in his usual vague way, 'Ah, you will find out in good time. Your trip in India is an adventure. Your trip into your incarnations will be yet another adventure.'

Finding a past-life therapist

Vikram couldn't have been more right. On my return to England I was determined to find a good therapist in past-life regression (PLR), which I had began to hear about as *the* tool to access your past existences. There was a buzz about this latest therapy and I had to try it because it really was at the forefront of spiritual exploration. For me, the concept of being able to access your past reality felt like being given an opportunity to walk into another dimension. It was mind-blowing.

But finding a PLR therapist proved to be much harder than I had envisaged. I searched through bookshops and magazines and I asked everyone I knew if they could recommend anyone who was experienced and genuine. Very few of my friends and acquaintances had even heard of PLR. I felt as if the universe was conspiring against me and I was forced to put the idea of having the therapy on the back burner.

When Greta was alive she had repeatedly told me to be patient. She had tried to help me learn this lesson and now I felt that the universe was making me wait too. Then I found a flyer tucked inside a New Age magazine. The flyer was advertising a workshop with a past-life regressionist called Denise Linn, who would be visiting London. Linn is a well-known author, lecturer, writer and healer. Twenty-two years ago, she even successfully regressed a room full of nearly 1,000 people in Australia.

I rubbed my hands together when I found the flyer and shouted out, 'Thank you, universe!' as I dialled the number immediately to book two places – one for myself and the other for my friend Terri. With my rabbiting on about PLR she was by now as keen as I was to discover this therapy.

On the day of the workshop it was swelteringly hot weather as we took our seats in the Royal Horticultural Halls and Conference Centre in London. There were nearly 500 participants in the massive hall, which was full of rows of seats and reminded me of a school assembly. I wondered how Denise could work with so many people at once. As I sat down I had an intense feeling of irritation. I couldn't explain where it came from but just at that moment a woman sat in front of me. I didn't give her a thought, yet the feeling of irritation increased and I had the strongest urge to just walk out. In my mind I was thinking, 'Don't be crazy – you've waited absolutely years for this and now it's arrived you want to run off.' I couldn't make any sense of how I felt or what was happening.

Just then Linn appeared on stage. The entire room fell silent as she smiled and said, 'Where you are sitting is no accident. So if you have any funny vibes from the people around you that's the reason why. You haven't met them before in your current life but you have known them in a past existence, and soon you'll find out just when and where that was and the details of your shared experience.'

She then asked alternate rows to stand up and turn around to face the row behind them, and I found myself facing a girl the same height and colouring as me. While Penny and I had the same hair and skin tone, I was 7 stone and a size 8 and she was at least 18 stone and a size 22. We looked the same but opposite.

My friend Terri was facing a girl who was the same height and colour, with dark hair, pale skin and freckles. But Terri was very glamorous, whereas this girl was frumpy. Again, this odd pairing was the same but also opposite in a bizarre way. Before anyone had time to speak to the person they were facing, Linn said, 'I'm going to take you all back to a past life before you have a chance to talk to the people I have linked you with today. You will find that you will see the same past life as this person.' I'll be honest, I couldn't quite believe what I was hearing and I thought, 'How an earth is she going to do that here?'

Next, soothing music filled the room and Linn asked us to close our eyes. We had to imagine a bridge over 'the ever-flowing river of time'. Linn's soothing voice made me feel incredibly calm, and then she said, 'As you step off the bridge you will step into a past life.' Immediately I saw myself in India. I was very poor and hungry. I was standing outside a house and inside, people were laughing and happy and I knew I wasn't allowed to enter. My logical mind told me, 'You're just seeing this because Vikram told you about a previous life in India.' But my gut reaction was different. This felt real in every part of my body. Before I had time to think any more about this short experience, Linn brought us back to the present moment and I was lost for words.

Quickly, we had to talk to our 'partner' opposite us and tell them what we had seen in the past life. Penny was happy to talk, and she told me, 'I saw us both in India. We were brother and sister. I was the boy and our father gave me everything and you nothing. He starved you, he wouldn't even let you inside the house.' I was so shaken by the words and the revelation from this complete stranger that I could hardly string together a response. I didn't even tell her what I had seen, I simply said, 'I saw something similar.' The synchronicity was astounding. It was almost too much to cope with because it was like fate poking me, whispering in my ear and nudging me in the back all at the same time.

We had a short break and my mind continued to race like a whirling dervish while I drank a cup of tea. Terri and I obviously felt the same because we both mumbled that it 'was amazing'. Then we fell silent. We had been friends so long we didn't need to fill the air with words.

Once we were back in the hall, Linn took us into another past life, but when she went through the relaxation techniques she said, 'This time, you will jump to a life that you most need to know about now.' I saw myself as a young boy of about thirteen. I was black, with really long arms and legs. I looked down at my slender limbs astonished, it felt so odd. I knew I was in North Africa, in Morocco, but I had no way of pinpointing the year. I then saw a knife come towards me and stab me in my abdomen. The next thing I knew I was floating out of my body and looking down at my lifeless form. I had died. There was nothing more to this life and I came out of the PLR myself.

On the way home Terri and I revealed our lives and tried to make sense of what we had seen. I had never done anything like this before, so it was hard for me to make sense of it all. For days I couldn't stop thinking about my regression. I wondered whether it had taken me a long time to find a regressionist because I hadn't been ready to hear the information earlier. Questions and answers jostled for space in my thoughts and I felt I needed some clarity. I needed to know where I was heading in my life – and why.

The next spiritual step

I tracked down a clairvoyant called Marie. Several of my friends had visited her and found her to be very accurate and discreet. I had never met her before and at my reading she shuffled her tarot cards, laid them down in front of me and then asked me to choose six. As I picked them out, she asked, 'Do you have a scar here?' She pointed to the exact point on my abdomen where a red line cut across me, a silent reminder of my earlier operation. 'Yes,' I told her. She said, 'You know we create scars in our current life to reflect wounds from past lives. You were stabbed right there in a past life.' I couldn't believe my ears. It had never occurred to me to connect the ugly scar on my abdomen with my past life as the Moroccan boy who was stabbed in exactly the same place. As Marie talked, it felt as if I was finally receiving some answers. I had certainly waited long enough, and I hoped I had proved to the universe I had learned the lesson of patience.

Marie then said, 'I can see you hypnotising people. You'll show them their past and their future lives.' Again, a message about past lives, but I had no idea what she meant about showing people the future – this was a bizarre concept to me.

As I left Marie's cottage and headed for the train station, I thought about her message. Hypnotherapy appealed to me. I had been obsessed with finding a past-life regressionist and then the session with Denise Linn had been so mind-blowing that it made me keen to explore the technique further. Training myself was the next natural step and the comment from Marie was the nudge I needed to point me in the right direction again.

Sometimes random comments, kind acts or even cruel words from strangers can act as a catalyst to push us gently in the right direction. As I stepped onto the platform at Slough Station I said to myself, 'I had better go and qualify in hypnotherapy then.' I had found the next step on my spiritual path.

Training to be a hypnotherapist

I immediately took to hypnotherapy and completed the six-month private diploma course in eight weeks. I practised on everyone who was happy to let me try out my fledgling skills. At first I mastered just relaxing people using basic breathing techniques and visualisation. Then I moved on to smokers. I was thrilled to find I could easily help people to kick the habit by focusing on the benefits of how fantastic their lives would be as nonsmokers. I directed them to imagine how they would no longer smell of smoke. They saw themselves opening their purses and wallets, which were bulging with money; and of course there were the added health benefits such as reducing the risk of developing cancer.

Following this success, I began working with people who were grappling with all kinds of issues such as weight loss, phobias, relationship problems and even lack of confidence. I still work in this area now, because the results are effective and quick and I gain such satisfaction in helping people to help themselves. But back then, once I had the tools of hypnotherapy I couldn't wait to begin working with past-life regression.

I developed a few regression techniques through trial and error and my training, and again I tried these methods out on my friends. I asked them to imagine themselves in a corridor of doors and to see one door standing out. When they walked through it they would step into a past life. Another technique was for my client to imagine sitting on a white fluffy cloud that was floating through time and stopping at the right moment. When they stepped off, they would step into a past life.

The first person I regressed was my friend Don, using the corridor technique. Immediately he was through the door he said, 'This is odd. My feet are warm.' He then said, 'It feels as if I'm standing in water.' He went on to describe in detail his daily life as a Greek fisherman. When Don came out of the regression he said, 'That was amazing. It felt like I was actually there.'

I had deliberately not told him about my own past lives in India and Morocco because I didn't want to lead him or plant any suggestive thoughts into his unconscious. However, I wasn't surprised to discover that we had shared the experience of a past life in Greece – we had probably known each other because souls often reincarnate in the same groups and play out life lessons and pay off karmic dues. I had discovered my own tragic Mediterranean life purely by accident and, as is sometimes the case, especially with a traumatic death, the memory came to the surface with no prompting because I was revisiting the scene of the crime.

Three months after finishing my own hypnotherapy training, I went on holiday to Rhodes in Greece. While I wandered around the town on the first day, I had the weirdest sensation. Everywhere I went I had a strange feeling of *déjà vu*. I knew the layout exactly of the town centre, and at every turn I predicted what would be around the corner, such as a little church. It was so odd. Trying to push it out of my mind, I spent the rest of the day lying on the beach. I dozed off but soon woke with a start. I suddenly sat up. It felt as if my throat had been cut. There was a sharp searing pain that took my breath away, and it was a real shock.

The sensation only lasted a few seconds, but I was still very shaken. I couldn't think what it was and was very confused. For the rest of the holiday I couldn't shake off the *déjà vu* either. Everything seemed so familiar, as if I were visiting a favourite holiday spot, even though I had never been there before in my life.

When I arrived back home, my best friend Terri, who had accompanied me to the Denise Linn workshop, said she had been for a one-to-one past-life regression while I was on holiday. She had been regressed the same day I had experienced the strange feeling on the beach. Terri told me, 'I saw us in Greece together. We were murdered. We had had our throats cut. It was so traumatic.'

All those miles away, I had glimpsed a previous existence at the same time as my friend and relived my death. It sounds mad, but that's the only explanation. We worked out the time difference and I was on the beach exactly when she was having the regression session. It was just the kind of event that, again, made me want to research past lives and hone my regression techniques.

Healing pain with past-life therapy

Thanks to practising on friends and my training, I was able to deliver quick results for my clients, and soon the phone was ringing with people who wanted to be regressed. Each past life was unique. Every person I took back in time gained something wonderful. They discovered previous past-life links with friends, family and partners who were part of the same soul family. The more you discover about your past lives, the more complete you will feel, almost as if you are finding missing pieces of the jigsaw. It will put you more in touch with the real you. It will explain aspects of yourself that you have never understood, such as finding it hard to get along with certain people or what seems like an irrational fear or phobia. As you become more in touch with yourself, your senses will heighten and your intuition will become more a natural part of your psyche.

Sometimes sessions unveiled the origins of an illness. Joe is a good example. He constantly had sore throats and in his regression he saw himself being hanged in medieval times for stealing food. Some people discovered a talent, such as Gary, who saw himself as a cowboy. Being inquisitive, he wanted to discover whether his natural ability in the saddle had transferred to this lifetime. He booked himself a riding lesson and discovered that as soon as he mounted a horse he could ride it. He told me later, 'Ah, now I know why I love baked beans!'

Other clients 'know' the countries they lived in and when, as well as their professions and hobbies, which explained talents they carried over into this life (such as those of Gary the cowboy). Each regression became a revelation and I loved it. When I'm working this way now, often I have glimpses in my mind's eye of what they're seeing, or at times I have a flash of the missing pieces for them, which makes it wonderful fun when we talk about it afterwards. Some people jumped from one life to another during their regression and saw a whole string of lives in just one session.

Regression and life's big questions

By visiting various lifetimes you find a theme or problem that has run through each of your lives. Many of my clients have found that, lifetime after lifetime, the same issues have occurred, causing them pain and distress. Rose came for a session with me because she had a terrible phobia about water. Even driving past a river or seeing the sea on television threw her into a panic. Our first session showed her as a sailor aboard a ship sinking in the middle of the ocean. All lives were lost. Then she jumped to another lifetime as a small boy who fell into a river while trying to reach a toy. In yet another lifetime she saw herself tied to a stool, being ducked into a river with the local townsfolk shouting, 'Witch, witch!' while she drowned. At the end of the session I helped Rose release her fear of water, which had accumulated through her previous lives and carried over into this one.

Often we find that relationships have also continued lifetime after lifetime, which is fine if the relationship is good. However, if it isn't positive and instead repeats hurt and anguish over and over, it can lead to a miserable and destructive experience in the here and now. Shannon was in a difficult relationship with Matt. They cared a great deal about each other, but Matt tried to control her. He made all the financial decisions and somehow it always ended up with her having no money in the bank while he had plenty. The strange thing was, she often jokingly called him 'the mad monk' because he had lost his hair in a perfect circle in the centre of his head.

During the session with me, Shannon saw herself in a monastery with Matt as her guardian. She was an orphan but came from a wealthy family. Her mother had died young and her father arranged for her to be cared for by the monks after his death. They would also be guardians to her and her money until she was old enough to make the decisions for herself. Shannon realised that they had simply repeated the pattern again in this lifetime, even though she was more than able to take care of her finances herself. At first they had a few disagreements, but after a while Matt stopped trying to control everything, which resulted in a much more balanced relationship.

Many people who are struggling with money in their current lifetimes have lived in poverty before and are simply recreating what is familiar. Sometimes people are trying to make up for what they see as bad behaviour in a previous life. One of my clients, Yvonne, is married to a wealthy man and she gave up her own lucrative career as an actress when she tied the knot. Yvonne came across as rather prim and so was stunned to find during our session that she had been a maid and a mistress to a great lord who kept her hidden in another part of his castle away from his wife. In her current life she waited on her husband hand and foot and realised that this was a habit from when she was a maid/mistress. She recognised her current husband as the lord from that lifetime!

During her session Yvonne spoke with an air of shame about her circumstances and in her current life she seemed to apologise for almost everything. By releasing this old pattern she went back to her career and became much more assertive.

Case study

Scraping by one Christmas left Janine with an unexplained fear of being poor, which haunted her until the issue was solved by past-life regression. The problem surfaced two years ago when she had a particularly rotten Christmas after the UK's Child Support Agency made a mistake and she had no money for presents.

'It broke my heart to rely on family to buy gifts for my seven-year-old daughter,' she says. 'The whole experience triggered a phobia about being poor. I found myself watching every penny. As a single mum, money's tight but I've never been on the breadline and I didn't need to turn into Scrooge. There was something strange about that Christmas too. I had a real feeling of *déjà vu* which didn't make sense and it unsettled me.'

So she booked a session of past-life regression, wondering if the answer to her fear could be found in a previous lifetime. 'As a reiki master I believe in reincarnation, and within seconds, after Anne used her relaxation techniques, I was in a light trance,' she explains. 'All she did was count down from 20 to one and then got me to imagine a corridor of doors. As I walked through the door I just knew I was a twenty-two-year-old American woman. I was wearing a blue dress and a white apron. I was standing in a big kitchen and it felt like it was around 1912. My duties were cleaning. The cook was always miserable.

'Anne directed me, "Move to a recent Christmas during this lifetime." The images were clear but only lasted a few seconds. I was with my husband John and our three children in our small house. There are no decorations – it's so poor and basic. We're always struggling financially.

'I feel frustrated at being so poor when I work so hard. Then it all makes sense – the memory of this life is still affecting me now. Anne replied, "You don't need to worry about being poor any more. In a previous life you were poor, that time and existence has gone forever. Leave this fear where it belongs in the past."

'Minutes later I came out of the trance. For days I felt refreshed, happy and positive. I've realised that my fears about money were dragging me down. But since the session I've beaten my phobia and I'm looking forward to a happy Christmas. It's funny, the less I've worried about the money, the more I seem to have in my pocket.

'Anne told me, "Think negatively and that's what you'll attract, be positive and your life will be full of joy." And I believe her.'

Top tips to gain the most from a regression

◆ Find a good regressionist by asking around friends rather than picking one out of the phone book or from the Internet.

◆ Be open-minded – it will probably not be what you expect.

◆ Do not try too hard, just let it happen.

◆ Don't worry if you do not 'see' anything. You may 'feel' or you may just simply 'know' the information depending on your dominant psychic sense or senses.

◆ Ask yourself what you need to learn from seeing this lifetime.

Discovering Your Primal Self

Before we leave the subject of delving into our dim and distant past, try this wonderful exercise for getting in touch with your primal self. I believe that in an earlier soul incarnation, you will have experienced a lifetime in which you were more primitive, more in tune with the earth and the universe. Your instincts were strong and your intuition sharp. Do the following visualisation to get back in touch with this aspect of yourself.

1. Feel yourself relaxing and imagine it's a sunny day and you are out in nature. Feel yourself sitting in a field with your back against a tree. Imagine you look up at the sky and watch the clouds floating by. You notice one of the clouds floating down and landing beside you. You sink into the cloud and feel its softness. It moulds itself perfectly to you.

2. Now feel the cloud, with you now on it, floating up into the air and backwards through time. Close your eyes and know that you are floating back to a lifetime where you lived a primitive life. You hunted, you listened to your dreams, you understood omens.

3. Allow the cloud to float down into that lifetime and relive that life. Notice how sharp your instincts are. Can you hear things at a distance? Do you notice omens? Do you have dreams and visions? Can you sense danger? Can you sense which path to take? Get in touch with all the abilities from this lifetime and keep them with you as you climb back on your cloud and float back to your present time.

From time to time tap into the feelings you had during the exercise and each time you do, they will become a part of you in your present life.

Discovering Future-Life Progression

As well as helping people with their problems, which, as you've gathered can sometimes be traced back to a past life, I was having other unexpected experiences with clients during PLR sessions. The first happened when I regressed a young woman called Fiona. Instead of floating back through time, Fiona actually jumped forward aeons into the future. She began talking about life on a spacecraft. At first I just thought she had a vivid imagination but for some reason I couldn't dismiss it. It all seemed very real and I had glimpsed some of the progression myself. I had seen flashes of a futuristic craft.

Fiona was a very down-to-earth girl who worked in a bank and she had visited me for one regression session previously. This regression – or should I say *progression*? – captured my imagination and I began searching for information about moving forward in time. I didn't even know what to call it. During my own research, I discovered some studies that had been carried out by the respected psychologist and hypnotherapist Dr Helen Wambach. Initially, she had been motivated by a desire to debunk reincarnation, beginning in the mid-1960s, and had conducted a ten-year survey of past-life recalls using hypnosis with 1,088 people. Wambach asked very specific questions about the time periods in which the subjects lived, the clothing, footwear, utensils, money, housing, etc, that they used or came into contact with in these lives.

She concluded that, with the exception of 11 subjects, all descriptions of clothing, footwear and utensils were consistent with historical records. Between 1980 and 1988, Wambach and her colleague, Dr Chet Snow, took 2,500 people into the future using deep-relaxation and trance techniques. The hypnotherapists were the first to stumble across the concept of progression after people undergoing PLR in their study jumped forward to future lives without any prompting.

After reading about Wambach and Snow's studies, I began my own work with Future-Life Progression, or FLP. I immediately realised it's very similar to PLR, but of course you travel into the future rather than the past. I believe it's a powerful tool for getting your life on track. How? It shows you how your current actions and thoughts will shape your future and design your destiny. Who will you be? What will you be doing? Where will you be and with whom? These are just some of the questions that can be answered.

As with PLR, I used trial and error to develop my own FLP methods and luckily I had many willing clients to practise my new skills on. I developed two methods of looking into the future which don't require years of training, just practice. Both techniques – which I call 'Esoteric TV' and 'The Corridor' – can be practised alone and are completely safe and simple to follow. I still use these methods today and have since taken hundreds of people into their own futures using this form of guided visualisation and light trance to help them find solutions to burning problems in their lives.

Just think about this. Imagine if you could see yourself in five years' time and could discover who you are in love with – or not – what friends are around you, where you are living and where you are working. You would have a strong snapshot of just how your life will be if you stay on your current course, what has worked and what hasn't. Using FLP, you tap into your Instant Intuition, which shows you which way to go. Your path will become clearer and you will have insight into the right direction for a required outcome. In your everyday life, you will instinctively know what helps to build the good things that you see during FLP and how to avoid the actions that create a negative result.

In the first exercise, I will show you how to move forward in time and actually see what you will be doing in five years, ten years and even 100 years from now, in your next lifetime – or whatever date you choose to view. I will also show you how to rewind and fast-forward your esoteric DVD player to get an immediate mini-movie of exactly what you need to know about the past or the future.

Before you begin your 'Esoteric TV' session, ask your Higher Self (simply think the words in your mind) to show you only what you need to know in order to improve your life. You do not want to see things that are upsetting – for example, an elderly aunt becoming ill or someone having a car crash. Things happen in life but there is no point in seeing these things unless there is something *you* can do to change it. Avoidance action is usually only possible if it is occurring in *your* life. With events concerning other people, these are their destiny and karma and you mustn't try to interfere. Only they can create their own future.

....

Esoteric TV

1. Imagine yourself in a beautiful room with a soft rich carpet, velvet curtains and subtle silk wallpaper. Your special room is so cosy and always at just the right temperature.

2. Notice in the corner the biggest, comfiest chair you have ever seen. The chair has warm, rich autumn colours. Imagine sitting in the chair and sinking right in. Feel the most relaxed you have ever felt, for you know that this is your private place and no-one can enter unless you invite them.

3. Now bring into view a huge plasma screen and DVD player, both in a solid-wood cabinet. Stop and think for a moment about what you want to know. Do you want to discover where you will be working in one year's time or who, if anyone, you will be dating? Do you want to see whether you will be happily married in five years' time or whether you will have children? Would you care to see if your next holiday will be fun or a washout? Or maybe look at next Christmas and see just who you will be having dinner with?

4. Focus on your esoteric TV screen and DVD player. Imagine reaching out and turning on the plasma screen. Now fast-forward the DVD machine to the allotted time, then focus on the television. What do you see? Allow the images to appear and take the first thought, feeling or image that comes to you. Allow the image to develop just like a photograph.

Remember, once you have seen the future *for you*, you can change it if you wish. You can make intelligent decisions such as, 'That career move looks great. Why wait five years? I'm going for it now.' Or, 'I can see he'll be an awful partner. I'm moving on right away.' Or even, 'I will be a superb guitar player, I will start taking lessons this week.'

Does 'Esoteric TV' always work?

I have included different exercises for progressing into the future because different methods work better for different people. Try them both and see which works better for you. Often, people mistakenly expect their past-life or future-life session to be like watching a movie. Some people do experience it in this way, but many simply catch glimpses in their mind's eye – a little like jumping up and peering over a wall. Others see nothing at all but get a strong feeling of where they are, and some have thought forms coming into their mind almost as if they were being read to.

In my offices in Berkshire, I've tested my FLP methods with stunning results, sometimes in a group and sometimes in one-to-one sessions. In a consultation setting it's always used for the particular person's life, but one friend, Dave, a former soldier who you will meet properly in the next chapter, went into the future using 'Esoteric TV' to discover new technological trends for travel, and he saw a red flying car! He said, 'It's like a little two-seater jump jet. It's brilliant, and it's got low environmental impacts.'

At the time we assumed this mode of transport would be decades away, because it seemed like something out of a sci-fi movie. But out of curiosity we looked on the Internet and found the prototype – just as Dave described. It's called the M400 Skycar and has been developed by Moller International. The makers are now entering the final stages of testing and recently their spokesman and general manager, Bruce Calkins, told me, 'Once satisfied with the preliminary tests we will schedule a date for a major demonstration flight.' Skycar already has 100 orders for models certified by the Federal Aviation Administration (FAA) in the USA, likely to cost $995,000 each. Now, was this a coincidence or did Dave really have a glimpse the future of transport? I know what my answer is to that question.

Case study

Beautician Caitlin used the 'Esoteric TV' technique to see if she would be better off financially within a few years. As she watched her future unfold on the television screen she had built in her mind, she told me, 'Wow, I'm so rich. I'm approaching some huge metal gates and there's a long drive with trees both sides and a massive house. It's wonderful.' Some time later Caitlin moved into her new salon, which happened to be inside an old manor house with a long drive and big metal gates. She told me, 'I glimpsed this place and presumed it was my home, so I'll just have to carry on working hard for a while yet.' In a later session Caitlin saw herself with a string of salons – and this time she made sure they were all hers.

In the second exercise, 'The Corridor', you will travel through time in your mind using a corridor of doors. It seemed obvious to me that, if doors worked so well to take people *back* in time, the same principle could take them forward. By travelling into the past, my clients have found answers to many issues such as why they have not reached their potential or why love has evaded them. By using the same method to move *forward* through time, with visualisation, you can find even more answers to problems about love, life, money, work and friendships.

The Corridor

1. Close your eyes and relax. Imagine you are standing in the middle of a long corridor when suddenly you notice there is something strange about it. You feel as if you are standing on a hill. You realise that the corridor slants upwards in front of you and downwards behind you.

2. On the wall next to you is a sign with an arrow pointing downwards, saying PAST, and an arrow pointing upwards that says FUTURE.

3. Notice that all along the corridor there are doors. Look up and down the corridor and see which door you are drawn to. One will have something about it, maybe a light underneath it or a sign on it – something that will draw you to it.

4. Go to that door and walk through. Take your immediate impression. Where are you? How old are you? How do you feel? What is happening?

5. Spend as long as you wish in this place. Then, when you are ready to leave, walk back through the door and close it behind you.

....

A regular client of mine, a hairdresser called Rachel, did the 'Esoteric TV' exercise during one of my workshops. Afterwards she told me, 'It doesn't make sense. I must have got mixed up with the past.' She saw herself clearly working at a salon where she was employed eight years ago. 'The weird thing is I hated the place because they treated me appallingly. Yet in the exercise I saw things going really well and my work was hugely successful. I looked so happy, I just can't understand it.'

A few months later, Rachel was approached by a businessman. He had just taken over the old salon where she used to work and he had heard she was a great stylist. He offered her a part of the salon. Within six months her turnover had trebled and she was very happy.

Another lady, Katie, who was thirty-five years old and had never had a boyfriend, came to me for a session. She was very lonely and had no idea how to flirt or chat up men. I took Katie into a future life and she had a wonderful husband. When she came out of the progression she said, 'Ah, I know how I have to act now to find a man!' Katie's mother died when she was young and she was brought up by her father. She told me, 'Somewhere along the line I didn't learn what other girls learn – stuff about boys and how to behave, how to show your feminine side. I just got on with helping my dad and keeping the home going when other girls were out meeting boys. I feel as if time's passed me by and now I would like to meet someone.'

I took her forward in time, where she found herself married to a lovely man. I asked her how she met him and how she behaved when she first met him. She told me, 'We had lots of things in common and so just struck up a conversation. It all happened quite naturally.' Katie became a lot more relaxed knowing that she would be happily married in her future. And, with the pressure taken off, she found that she could relate to men more easily – and she did find her dream man.

The knock-on effects

As well as seeing the future, something else began to happen among my clients, something almost magical. Things that they had seen – for instance, a new business or meeting their soulmate – began to occur much sooner than in the timeline they reported in the sessions. It was as if seeing something brought it into their present consciousness. Sheila is a good case to illustrate what I mean about timelines. She was forty-three years old and had been regularly beaten up by her drunken husband George for the past 20 years. He controlled and dominated the whole family and Sheila and the children were terrified of him. She came to me to see if at some point in her future she would have escaped from George.

I took her forward five years and she still saw herself miserable – and by this time he was worse. She was agitated but I reassured her that we can change the future if we wish. I then took her forward ten years from her present time. The hard look on her face that she had worn since her arrival was replaced by a soft, warm smile as she saw herself happy and living in a new house without him. In fact, she had no idea where he was or what he was doing. Glowing, she told me, 'At least I know one day I'll have some peace.'

I told her that this would probably now happen sooner. Sheila was astonished and told me, 'But I've seen I will be free in ten years.' I explained to her that once we've brought something into our conscious we can make it happen sooner, but I could see she didn't really believe me. So I told her, 'Let me take you back to the five-year point. I bet it looks different now.'

Sheila looked at me dubiously and as I took her forward something told me to take her to just the two-and-a-half-year mark. I did so and at that point a broad smile beamed across her face and she said, 'Ooh, I have a nice new man and there's no sign of my husband.' Six months after her session, Sheila came back to tell me she had left George. Within 12 months of our first session, she had met and moved in with her new, gentle and kind man.

I'm pleased to say that I have numerous other success stories of people changing their lives following FLP. Unlike with past lives, I haven't had any negative experiences in which people recall disturbing incidents. I believe this to be the case because your Higher Self is showing you the best you can be in this incarnation. The few people I am aware of who have used FLP have mainly worked with big groups and they have uncovered incredible information, but working on a one-to-one basis is special. There will be more information about this in my next book, but each and every person I have taken forward has changed.

The best way I can describe the effects of the therapy is to say that people seem more evolved, more aware of their life purpose. I don't think the future is set at all and we all have the free will to change our destiny. Put it like this: if you were to book a holiday and suddenly war broke out, you would cancel it and go somewhere else. At any time we are only seeing one of a number of possible futures (maybe infinite) which fate and destiny have crafted for us. FLP works on the same principle. I take clients into the future, using my tried and tested methods, and, if they don't like what they see – their karma – then they know they need to change their lives now. I believe karma is not only actions but thoughts, words and any intention.

Karma shapes our destiny. With this therapy, you've the power to change your karma because you can see where you'll be heading if you stay on a particular path. After all, we all have the power to choose the type of life we lead and this is one of life's great secrets – we control and manifest our own future.

I can also tell you from my heart that my work with FLP has made me very optimistic about the world and the human race and where we are heading. I have seen aeons into the future and it looks pretty good to me. I've trained in many areas – hypnotherapy, psychotherapy, thought-field therapy and NLP (Neuro-Linguistic Programming). Although all produce good results, I feel FLP to be the most powerful tool I've ever used in my work and it came about due to bizarre synchronicity. But as you know, in reality there is nothing coincidental about coincidence.

CHAPTER 6
Boosting Your Instant Intuition

One of my offices is near Windsor and it's not uncommon for me to see celebrities and ladies who lunch in the same afternoon. However, I was surprised when a soldier came for a psychic consultation, then another and another. While Greta was alive I had never done a reading for anyone from the Forces. I had expected military men to be sceptical but actually the reverse was true.

To this day I have not met a soldier, or a policeman or -woman, who doesn't use his or her sixth sense. Every last one of them has woken up and known something big was going to happen that day or has just 'known' danger was around the corner. This has made me realise that Instant Intuition isn't a gift for the chosen few but it is a birthright. For each and every one of us, this skill is waiting to be awakened. Once you tap in, you can do mind-blowing things with it if you dare to try – which was always Greta's message.

Jungle consciousness

One day, after I had given him a reading, I asked Dave, an ex-paratrooper, if it was normal for soldiers to be psychic and to rely on their intuitive powers. 'Yes,' he replied. 'Years ago it wasn't really talked about but now it's almost taken for granted in the Army. No-one stands with his hand on his forehead saying, "Hang on lads, I'm having a premonition." You just know something.'

Steve, who now works in security, often in war zones, told me he regularly used his instincts, his intuition, while he was in the Army. 'We were in Belize in the jungle for six months and I'm a bad map reader, so often I would use my instincts,' he explained.

I asked him, 'Did you get lost in the jungle? That must be terrifying.'

Steve replied, 'We never talk about getting lost in the Army: we call it "being geographically embarrassed". Anyway, I would just know the way back and I would tell the lads, "It's this direction." They would never question how I knew the way, and neither would I.'

On another occasion, I was chatting to Dave and I wondered whether he ever had premonitions. He said, 'For me, I don't wake up and know something will be happening that day: I know just beforehand. If the ESP [extrasensory perception] kicked in too early it wouldn't be as useful.'

His comment about timing made sense to me. It's common for most people to get a sudden gut feeling and react, but if the feeling comes too early they usually talk themselves out of it — unless they are using their Instant Intuition. The feeling Dave refers to is a spiritual nudge which comes just when we need it.

I wondered where Dave felt that this ESP information came from and he said it originated from a part of his brain that's normally dormant. He explained when I pressed him for more detail, 'My brain feels like a house where there's one room which isn't used very often. I can't point to my head and tell you exactly where this spot is but I know it's in there and it turns itself on at crucial moments. It's like an empty room, then suddenly the light goes on.' I then asked him something I really wanted to know: 'Do the Army give you any training in how to boost your intuition?' His answered fascinated me. I will let him tell you in his own words.

He said, 'Yes, in the Special Services they call the training "jungle consciousness". They take us into the jungle and we observe everything around us. We're taught that if someone is searching for us and they look in the direction of, say, the bush where we're hiding behind, even though they can't see us, we're told to look away. We must not look at the eyes of the enemy, otherwise we would make a psychic connection and they would then "know" our hiding place.' According to Dave, the Army even use the words *psychic connection* to explain their methods during training.

Dave told me that to fine-tune his jungle consciousness – in short, to boost his intuitive skills – the Army kept him and his select regiment there for two weeks, which is the routine length of time to practise this part of training. 'It takes from a week to ten days for the jungle consciousness to kick in,' he explains. 'Some people think this is a harsh and unnecessary part of training, but really you couldn't do it for any less time. After ten days outside and living on your wits you're in animal mode. When you first arrive your senses are all over the place.

There's so much noise you feel bombarded and can't distinguish one sound from another. But after a while you begin to home in, and the noise levels out. You begin to know, to sense, the difference between the wind rustling the trees and a predator rustling them. It's a heightened state of awareness. You use no energy – you stop and focus. There could be a snake a mile away and the same colour as the jungle, yet you would see it. Honestly, it would stand out over and above all the thousands of things in your view. You become a super-predator yourself.'

Search mode

The soldiers are great fun and I've enjoyed quite a few nights in the pub with them, chewing over everything from world events to remote viewing (RV) – which I'll be talking about soon. One thing I've noticed from spending time with these military men is that their Instant Intuition is always switched on and ready, thanks to their training. They are fascinating to watch because there's something in them that is constantly filtering or scanning for information for anything that just isn't right. Their sense of danger is red-hot. I often joke with them saying, 'I bet you sleep with one eye open.' And from watching them I've developed a technique I call *search mode*.

I may be sitting in a traffic jam or in a relative's house, or I may be queuing in the greengrocer's. But rather than clock-watch, I will be tapping in and asking myself, 'Is there anything coming up I should know about now?' Some of my best predictions have also come from when I have been in the dentist's or doctor's waiting room practising search mode. For me, it acts as a quick booster to my Instant Intuition. Think of it as a pro tennis player practising their best return shot for the odd five minutes every day. The champion already knows they can hit a killer ball, but they can always be that little bit better. Search mode boosts your intuitive skills because it will get you into the habit of using your sixth sense all the time. It will keep your Instant Intuition on alert so that things that would normally go unnoticed will be brought to your attention – but only if you need to know. You will pick out the one piece of information that you need at that moment.

In search mode you will find information that most people miss, such as a cashier who is short-changing people. You will notice their eyes dart about to make sure no-one sees what they're doing or the fact that they don't count out the change. You may 'sense' a car travelling too fast along a busy road where children are about, and pull one child back in the nick of time. One of my clients, Doreen, was at a busy road with three lanes of traffic and says, 'For some reason I didn't step out onto the crossing, even though the green man came up. A split-second uneasy feeling stopped me and immediately afterwards a car sped through the red light. If I had been on the crossing I would have been hit at 80 miles an hour.' What saved her? Her boosted Instant Intuition, which was switched on and working.

Some years ago I arrived late at night in a holiday resort called Altinkum in Turkey. I dropped my bags in my room and went for a walk to explore the noisy busy streets. As I entered the town square I scanned the area. My instincts told me to look up and to my right. As I did so, a girl on the balcony of a nightclub looked down and for some reason, as we caught sight of each other we laughed. Later, we bumped into each other again in the club and ended up chatting. Her name was Sharon. She had gone to Turkey to get over the tragic death of her partner and she had taken a job in a nightclub. Ever since fate, and search mode, brought us together, we have kept in touch.

Going into search mode helps us filter out what we don't need and takes us to the incidents or people who are meant to enter our reality. The square in Altinkum was packed with people and filled with bright lights, noise and activity. There are clubs, bars and restaurants all competing for customers, and there are the excited holidaymakers. If I had stopped to look and listen I would not have seen Sharon. It was my psychic senses that guided me to look up and see her.

On another occasion I visited a friend's West End nightclub. It was his birthday and the place was packed. As always, I scanned the room and was drawn to a man standing quietly with a group of people. He seemed to be listening to them attentively. At that moment I caught a glimpse of him. There was something different about this person. I wasn't sure what, but I was curious to find out. At that moment my friend the club owner appeared and said, 'Anne, you must meet my colleague. We're doing some business together.' He took me straight to the gentleman and introduced me as his 'business psychic'.

The man turned out to be one of the most innovative people alive today. He was a billionaire by his early 30s, yet few people would know who he was if they walked past him in the street – and that's how he likes it. He is a deeply spiritual man who has never been influenced by money and I believe I was meant to meet him.

You can easily develop your own search mode and benefit from the information you receive. Remember, don't try too hard, as I used to when I was little. Let it flow.

Making an Impression

In a room full of people and noise, your mind is being bombarded with a million different things. The brain has its own natural filtering system. If you were aware of everything within your vision you would go crazy. This exercise simply heightens the filtering system so that what you need to know comes to the surface.

The next time you arrive at an event, or function, just scan the room with your eyes. Don't look at anyone directly – in fact, direct your eyes above their heads and you will find that you will pick up impressions.

Don't try too hard – just allow your impressions to guide you. What do you feel? Who are you drawn to? Who do you feel wary of? Do not censor – simply take the impressions and trust them.

There will be people who feel really good fun and there will be others who feel snobbish, aloof or annoying. People talk about first impressions and usually these are based only on appearances. But if you take the first impression using your intuition, you will pick up the person's subtle vibrations, their inner being and what you really need to know about them to help you to decide how to interact with them.

Search mode doesn't have to be done in an actual place, or in the same room as someone. Often I take a few minutes while I'm in my office or waiting in the supermarket queue to focus on a friend or acquaintance. I build up a picture of them in my mind and I look to see where they are and what they are doing. The next day I will call them up and ask, 'So what did you do yesterday?' With people I know very well, I will ask them, 'So how did the date go last night?' or, 'You must be tired today, you were out very late for a weekday.' They find it hilarious that they can't hide anything from me.

My friend Jenny's partner, Wayne, told me, 'It must be terrible to have a girlfriend like you. You know everything they're up to.'

I told him, 'Only if they were up to things they shouldn't be. Perhaps I should teach your girlfriend a few of my methods.' Wayne looked rather pale when I left their house.

Soul groups

My soldier friends, who had originally come for tarot readings, also started to come for past-life regressions. They proved to be great hypnotic subjects and were very keen to learn all they could about their former lives. They experienced lifetime after lifetime as warriors, sometimes fighting together, sometimes against each other. They had no trouble recognising one another, and other people, from their lives now. Their regressions were never dull and they are amazing to work with because they are disciplined and focused and always turn up on time.

Steve, a former Scots Guard, had so many PLR sessions with me that he became confident in the process and began regressing army colleagues himself. Steve also regressed me and a friend we have in common, Dave, the ex-paratrooper we met earlier, many times. During the sessions we often saw ourselves together in a number of different lives. We had all known each other in numerous previous existences, which explained the easy rapport and the trust that enabled everyone to go under so quickly.

A lifetime that stood out particularly was one Dave saw when he was regressed by Steve. He saw me in a Native American existence and, keen to find out more, Steve regressed me without revealing any details of Dave's vision. As soon as Steve said the words, 'You have now entered a past life', I saw myself sitting outside a tepee cross-legged. I knew I was an American Indian medicine woman.

Suddenly, I was aware of the thunder of hooves and a rival tribe charged through the camp. I felt an impact and knew a tomahawk had been thrown at my head. I flinched as the weapon made its impact. I want to emphasise that at no stage did I feel any pain or feel any distress. The next thing I knew, it was a later time in that lifetime and I was surprisingly alive, albeit with a big dent in my head. My instincts told me that the attacker was one of my solider friends. Later they told me they had both seen the very same scene, but neither was willing to tell me which one of them had thrown the tomahawk!

Our experiences together during our past-life sessions illustrate the fact that we belong to the same soul group. Every single person has a soul group they are linked to and with each incarnation members of the same soul groups meet again and again to learn spiritual lessons and hopefully grow together. Just recently I visited an iridologist called Janet in another part of the country. She began talking about a nutritionist she knew who lived in Cornwall. Amazed, I told her, 'I know Roger. He's given me advice over the telephone.'

A little later, Janet mentioned that it would be good for me to have some Bowen technique, a form of gentle manipulation of the body that helps you to regain balance. I told Janet there was a good chap near to me called Stuart, who was skilled in this therapy. She replied, 'Oh, I know him.' I had never been to her area before and she had never been to mine, but somehow we are in the same soul group and therefore have come across the same people. You will know if someone is in the same soul group as you. You will have an instant feeling of familiarity as soon as you meet, or you may have a strong feeling of wanting to get to know them or even feel as if there's unfinished business. Being aware of your soul group, and connections with other people, is yet another way of boosting your Instant Intuition and the messages it sends you. Notice when you feel a connection with another person. There is bound to be some link – even if you have just arrived in a strange country and never had any connection to the place. If there is something familiar about something or someone, explore it. You never know what you might find.

Remote viewing

One night in the pub Steve the soldier asked me, 'Why do you think we've ended up in the same soul group? Is there something we need to be doing?' I told him I was sure there was a reason and added that somehow their military and my spiritual backgrounds had been brought together this time around for a reason. But I had no idea what. I told Steve, 'The only thing I can think of is remote viewing. But all the training I've heard of has been very expensive and is available either in America, Australia or Hawaii.'

Steve said, 'Wouldn't it be amazing if we could learn how to do it?'

I trusted the process and put the thought out to the universe. Three days later, I received an invitation to train with Lee James Heather, a top remote-viewing trainer, in London. This was the first RV workshop that I was aware of in the UK. I had no idea what we would gain from it but somehow I knew it was the next step along our path. Steve often got frustrated by not knowing the end result of the journey, but often we know only the very next step. It's like driving along a dark, long road with our headlights on: we can see only the next hundred yards at any given time, yet our journey may be of hundreds of miles.

The RV training that I received in 2002 was not at all what I expected. I'm used to using my EET to 'feel' or to build pictures in my mind, or experiencing things in great detail as with my FLP methods, which now you will be familiar with and should be practising in your daily life. RV, however, was a whole new ball game.

We looked quite an odd bunch as we arrived at the training office in Fulham, London. There were three big, strong army men and me. The men made straight for the desk at the front of the room immediately in front of our trainer, Lee. They all stared intently at him, waiting for him to impart his knowledge. Their concentration was total and a lesser man not used to talking to groups would have been intimidated. Lee explained to us, 'RV is not a psychic gift. In fact, anyone can remote-view and it's a skill like any other which you can learn. You simply need to know the techniques, then practise them.'

He explained that remote viewers are given a reference connecting them to the object they are to view. For example, I may decide the target is the plush chair by the newspaper rack in the foyer of the Dorchester Hotel in London. This object will be given a reference number.

The number is not a grid reference, but simply a reference given to the object. However, once the reference has been given, that information is 'out there' for remote viewers to pick up on. I know this sounds amazing but this has been proven to work over and over again. The reference number gives the remote viewer a link to the object. So we could give the Dorchester chair the reference C-145. Once we've allocated that reference, we give this code to the remote viewer.

Now there are a number of ways of remote viewing and I've experimented with numerous ones since this initial training, but I've found Lee's method to be the most effective. He taught us to use symbols, such as a wavy line to represent water, and to ask split-second questions and use the split-second responses. Lee would give us the reference and at that very moment we were to use a symbol to say whether this was a manmade structure or something natural. He would then fire the questions at us, 'Is it outside or inside? Large or small? Synthetic or natural?' We would write a symbol for each answer in less than a second.

Lee explained that the key was to put down our impression before we had time to think or try to guess. It took me a little while to adjust because, although I practise Instant Intuition, I usually focus and concentrate for several moments. Often I do instantly know something and usually I have a picture in my mind, but not always, and it can take a few minutes to build up an image. Lee was adamant, however, that we had to go with our instant response.

Our first target was a range of mountains. Steve put down symbols for outside, big and natural. I put down the symbol for stone. Finally, we were to draw a very quick picture. Steve drew a range of mountains, as did I with no cross-reference. Throughout the rest of the afternoon we picked up 'targets' such as the Eiffel Tower and then an Egyptian pyramid. The lads were impressed by their results and I could see easily why the CIA had spent cash on carrying out complicated research into RV's effectiveness at places such as the Monroe Institute in Virginia, an organisation dedicated to exploring human consciousness.

....

Remote Viewing

Try this simple RV exercise with a friend.

Ask the 'monitor' to find several pictures of places and put them into separate sealed envelopes. (The monitor is the person who guides the remote viewer. They know what is in the envelopes, or what the target is, and often set the task.) Make sure nothing can be seen from the outside. Then they need to number each envelope.

It's a good idea to make the pictures of things you can clearly see and describe, such as a mountain range, Ayers Rock, or Big Ben. Also, make the pictures very different from each other.

Find yourself somewhere quiet to work, preferably with not too many things in view. We used to do this in my office boardroom. It had nothing in it other than a long table, chair and plain white walls. If this is not possible, try to be facing a plain wall.

Now place in front of you a pen and several pieces of paper. Write your name in the top right-hand corner, and the date and time in the top left-hand corner. Choose one of the envelopes. Write 'Target' in the top centre of the paper, followed by the number on the envelope.

As soon as you write the target number, write down or draw every impression that comes to you. Really allow the ideas to flow. Most people find it best to sketch what comes to mind, followed by words. You may sketch a big building or a tree; you may have no idea what it is but just feel that it is a certain shape. You may write words such as 'rain', 'big', 'dark', 'outside' or 'inside', or a phrase such as 'building many people'. Also make a note if you have any feelings or any other impressions.

Don't worry about whether it makes sense or not – very often it doesn't until you find out the target. Some people prefer to have six images and decide which one to view with the throw of a dice.

Another method, which is an interesting and fun way to work, is to tell a friend to go to a location of their choice at a particular time. At the appointed hour, draw and write any impressions that come to you. They may be in a children's park, or a train station or anywhere that is quite distinctive.

....

The psychic spy

F. Holmes 'Skip' Atwater is a former clairvoyant spy and captain in the US Army, who trained and recruited RVs for the Stargate programme, one of a number of remote-viewing exercises carried out by the CIA. He says, 'In essence, the remote viewer must let their mind go and trust the information which comes back without analysing it. Analysing the data was found to cause confusion.'

Some of the real targets against which RVs were employed for army intelligence included locating hostages, a kidnapped Army general in Italy, pinpointing drug shipments in Central America and many other sensitive situations.

'In fact, orders were taken from US Army installations all over the world. As people moved jobs, they took the knowledge of our existence and operations with them. We took tasks from all the intelligence services including the Central Intelligence Agency (CIA), Drug Enforcement Agency (DEA), and the Federal Bureau of Investigation (FBI),' he explains.

'We identified KGB spies, located Soviet weapons and technologies such as a nuclear submarine in 1979, helped find lost Scud missiles in the first Gulf War and plutonium in North Korea in 1994. Over the duration of the programme there were some significant hits – even to the extent of personnel being awarded military commendations. We had a success rate of 47 per cent rated by the tasking agencies as being of intelligence value.'

But the task that Atwater feels was Star Gate's biggest counter intelligence coup involved a Russian submarine in the eighties. The US knew the Russians were up to something as they'd been spying on the Severodinsk Shipyard, in Siberia, using a high resolution satellite.

'A lot of material was going into the shipyard,' recalls Atwater. 'US intelligence knew the Russians were building something big – but what?

'Star Gate was assigned to find out what was going on. Neither myself, (I was the monitor for the task) nor the RV were given any information other than the geographical co-ordinates.

'In the first session, the RV immediately picked up that it was a very cold, snowy area. Then the next set of images he saw was men welding the framework of a large grey construction.

'We went back to the National Security Council, who'd given us the task, and they said: "You're on target, find out more".

'In the next and final session, the remote viewer went into the future and saw a large flat-nosed submarine with missiles which were cantered forward. At the time, this was very important information as the subs used by the USSR had until then had to stop to fire missiles.

'The new technology meant the Soviet subs would be able to fire while moving. Then, the RV went forward again in time to find out the launch date of the submarine.

'He saw tractors digging a huge trench – which was later flooded – and the sub going out to sea. But due to our successful RV exercise, US intelligence had a satellite taking pictures the moment it was launched.'

At that time, the Oscar Class Submarine, as it became known, was the largest submarine built by the Russians. The information provided by Star Gate's RV was priceless.

Atwater adds, 'After my retirement from the Army in February 1988, where I reached the rank of captain, I took up the post of research director at the Monroe Institute. (Robert Monroe, 1915–1995, was the pioneer in the investigation of out-of-body experiences (OBEs) and the author of the groundbreaking book entitled *Journeys Out of the Body*. The Monroe Institute is a non-profit research organisation dedicated to the exploration of human consciousness.) Now I teach members of the public how to remote-view. The technique can be used for tasks like medical diagnosis, business projections, finding lost children and early-warning systems for natural disasters. My own view on RV and what I've seen is that all that exists is the present. What we call the past is information and what we call the future is formed by the laws of probability, intent-consciousness and present activities. In short, the past, present and future appear to exist at the same time in a multidimensional reality.

'In another decade or two, when the scientific community, which has so far done everything to discredit remote viewing, finally wakes up and the reality of these phenomena sink in, the way we look at the world will begin to change for ever. Humanity might then take its next big leap in consciousness.'

Although RV is not carried out in a science lab, I still find the following anecdote from Russell Targ's book *Limitless Mind* fascinating. In it, Targ tells the story of when he met the renowned energy healer Barbara Brennan, who wrote the seminal *Hands of Light*. Brennan has her own healing school in South Florida in the USA, where she teaches her students to see and feel a person's flow of chi (the life force in Chinese medicine and philosophy) and even to recognise imbalances in the energy field. For a spiritual worker, Barbara is unusual because she was a physicist at NASA, where she studied the reflection of solar light from Earth. Her scientific knowledge has given her the skills to describe the energy field in great detail and with unprecedented accuracy and expertise.

Targ himself is a renowned remote viewer and they were fascinated by each other's work and were delighted to meet each other in New York. Brennan hid a small object in his hotel bathroom and asked Targ to 'see' it using his remote-viewing skills. Targ then described it as a small red object with spikes sticking out of it. It was a red hairbrush. As Targ remotely viewed the object from his room, the former NASA scientist sat nearby and watched a beam of light flowing from Targ in the direction of the unidentified target. Amazing! For me, this story illustrates how energy really does emanate from our mind and plays a major part in our development and success with regard to what I call Instant Intuition.

The expert's view

The writer, philosopher and renowned paranormal investigator Colin Wilson has investigated everything from UFO abductions to poltergeist hauntings. He gave his view on remote viewing especially for the readers of *Instant Intuition*. Wilson believes time travelling is possible, and says, 'Scientific investigation has shown that Monroe's claims can be substantiated in the laboratory. Most people can learn the techniques of out-of-the-body experiences in a fairly short time. I first heard about remote viewing from Ingo Swann [an artist who helped to develop the process of RV at Stanford University with CIA money], who I met while researching a feature. He described experiments where he'd had to leave his body and identify various targets during training for the CIA.'

Wilson adds, 'I went to the Monroe Institute myself to check out remote viewing in 1997. I spent an hour in a black room but nothing happened. I didn't have an amazing experience. But that's not to say time travel, remote viewing, or whatever you want to call it doesn't exist. There are lots of examples of people who have conducted experiments outside of the military arena. The scientists Charles Tart, Robert Jahn and Brenda Dunn are well known for their vigorous scientific tests in this field. They've discovered that the most important aspect for remote viewing to work is for the subject to be relaxed. I believe that primitive people had these psychic powers, such as being able to RV, and that animals possess them now, which is how they know when their owner is coming home. But, over the millennia, we've got rid of the faculty as in a modern society we don't need it. Psychics, however, still have these abilities and are tapping into an ancient skill and accessing other dimensions.'

Other cultures, such as the Amazon Indians, acknowledge these invisible worlds, which Wilson believes operate at a higher vibration. They exist in the same space, but we live life wearing sunglasses and see only a small part of reality.

'Intuition is by far the most important faculty we possess.'

Colin Wilson

Remote viewing or future life progression?

While initially remote viewing and future-life progression (see Chapter 5) may appear to be the same practice, they are very different. RV appears to rely on symbols and works better with specific events that have already occurred, such as a plane crash. This is the reason why governments have been keen to utilise RV, because it's the perfect way to keep an eye on the enemy and see just what they are up to. It's been used, according to ex-military RVs, to find enemy ammunition dumps and discover the location of prisoners. It's great for looking at a particular place and to 'see' what is happening there.

RV also needs a trained person called an 'interviewer' or 'monitor' to guide you – unless you are very experienced. It also gives a snapshot of information. The technique can take many hours to learn, and even experts often describe feeling utterly exhausted after their session.

With FLP, like PLR, you're 'there' in the moment experiencing it, feeling it and connecting with the emotions. The information is more intense and lasts longer with no after effects. Also, FLP can be used effectively for a one-to-one personal experience about *you*, whereas RV tends to give better information for 'incidents'. You can do FLP by yourself. It's quick, simple and safe, and doesn't require hours of training at a top-secret military camp! So, while I value the experience of my RV training, I prefer working with FLP rather than RV to boost your Instant Intuition and to help you find the answers to life's important questions. For my purposes, I prefer FLP because I like to work with my clients either in a one-to-one session or in a group to help them see how their life has developed in the future. Most people want to know where they will be living and who they will be living with, and how their career is panning out, and the therapy can provide the answers. Try both methods and see which suits you better.

For many of you, the workplace is a place where you can now put into practice your strengthened intuition skills. We will be looking at how you can do this in the next chapter.

CHAPTER 7
Using Your Gut Instinct at Work

It's funny how we can meet one person and this can lead to a cascade of events that we could never have imagined. I often think life is similar to a game I used to play as a child. You spend ages setting up the lines of dominoes, like a miniature black-and-white Stonehenge, and you wait in anticipation to push the first one thinking you are in control. Then the dog comes in or a draft blows and the element of surprise takes over as one domino topples, causing a knock-on effect you can't do anything about – except sit back and watch. Thankfully, in life the end result isn't ruins but usually a new direction.

My involvement with the world of business, which is now a major part of my work, began with one such seemingly everyday event that had a knock-on effect. A young sales assistant called Alison came to see me for a reading. With the aid of my tarot cards I looked at her love life and the two men she had to choose between. I looked at her home life and the problems she had with her alcoholic mother, and I then examined her work. I told her, 'You'll soon be leaving your current job to go somewhere new.' This surprised Alison but, because the rest of the reading made so much sense, the young woman said she would keep it in mind.

Alison went back to the shop where she worked and, as you can imagine, the girls all asked, 'What did the psychic say?' She told me later they were quite intrigued because none of them had ever had a reading. One by one, each of the girls came to see me and every time I told them, 'You'll soon be leaving your place of work.'

I had no idea they all worked at the same shop, because I see so many people and each reading is fresh. Once I've finished a consultation I clear it from my mind, so it was a surprise to me when their boss Karen turned up at my office. She asked bluntly, 'What are you doing to my shop? You've told all my staff they're leaving.' I suggested to Karen that we look at her cards and, lo and behold, the tarot spread also showed *she* was moving on, which she pooh-poohed. Three months later, the shop closed down. The owner of the property had sold the building to a developer.

This experience was the beginning of a new business trend and the domino effect pushed me in yet another new direction. One person would come for a reading, followed by the rest of their colleagues, and finally the boss would appear at my door, intrigued and occasionally with a sneer. The sneering cynics usually sat down and said something like, 'I bet you won't be able to tell *me* anything.' I love these bosses. Usually all I need to do is tell them one little thing, maybe a secret dream they have or a problem from their past, and they are hooked. I love watching them sit back with their arms and legs firmly crossed, scared to twitch an eyebrow in case they give something away. But gradually they unfold, then lean forward, and in the end I have a job to get rid of them.

Many bosses came along open-minded, especially if things I had told the staff about the company rang true with what they already knew but were not revealing for a number of reasons. A director of a major airline came to see me and said, 'Several of my staff have been for readings. You've told them our firm will be going through major restructuring because we'll be buying another airline. Please don't tell anyone. We're about to take over an airline and if this news leaks out it could affect the stock market and our bid.' Of course I kept quiet and I certainly didn't buy any shares – I didn't want the fraud squad on my doorstep.

As I began to deal with more people who came for advice about their businesses, I found I could accurately 'feel' how the company was doing. Big cars started pulling up outside my little office in Slough, much to the astonishment of the other people in the building. Once in my private office, I would sit with the head of a global corporation and give them a rundown of just what was happening in their company and what was likely to take place in the future. Those at the top of the corporate ladder, or slippery pole, depending on your viewpoint, were intrigued and several called me their 'Secret Weapon'.

Is your boss psychic?

After a while, I began to notice a pattern emerging. The chairmen and directors would be open-minded but also cautious, while those in lower to middle management were less likely to come for a consultation. I wondered whether the people at the top were more intuitive so set about finding out if anyone had done any studies. What I discovered astounded me. There was little academic research in this area but I did find some nuggets.

The American parapsychologist Dr Douglas Dean and engineer John Mihalasky, an industrial management professor at the New Jersey Institute of Technology in America, spent over ten years in the seventies studying the predictive abilities of chief executives and how well their companies performed. One of their studies involved asking executives to predict a 100-digit number that would subsequently be chosen randomly by a computer between two hours and two years later. They found that the exceptionally higher-performing executives had above-average precognitive abilities. They also unveiled certain character traits in these individuals – they were fast-moving, dynamic people while the lower performers were more laid-back individuals.

In El Paso, Professor Weston Agor, of the University of Texas, conducted a study of 2,000 managers from a variety of backgrounds. He gave them 27 multiple-choice questions that, when answered, would give him an insight into their levels of intuition. His research found that the higher-level managers were more intuitive than the lower-level managers.

In his next test, he gave the top scorers a more specific questionnaire on how they used their intuition. In their answers they spoke of using their 'gut feelings' and trusting 'a sudden feeling of enthusiasm' or 'a feeling of calmness' when they made a particular choice they knew to be the right one. Agor asked the executives if they talked about their hunches and using intuition to make business decisions with their colleagues. The majority didn't. Personally, I've come to the conclusion that, while many bosses might not think of themselves as 'psychic', they certainly rely on their gut reaction more than people below them in the work hierarchy. I also believe senior executives are more open-minded to new or unusual ideas or at least willing to have a look. You may be interested to know that Agor discovered that those stuck at the lower levels relied on statistics and information far more than their own 'feelings' and were less likely to take risks.

> 'Experience taught me a few things. One is to listen to your gut, no matter how good something sounds on paper.'
>
> Donald Trump

Playing the stock market using intuition

Stock market trader Greg Secker has an impressive background. By the age of 24 he was made the youngest ever vice-president and head of online trading for Mellon Capital Corporation in the United States. This company was voted America's most admired company by *Fortune* magazine.

In 1997, he was responsible for creating one of the first global online dealing businesses supporting a money-market business that turned over billions on a daily basis. His training company, Knowledge to Action Ltd, is the only one of its kind to be approved by the Financial Services Authority (FSA). He is the only trader to publish his dealings and results weekly online – and he uses his intuition on a daily basis in his work.

Greg says, 'When I first began investing it was more like

gambling, then I began to use systems. The systems felt uncomfortable because they didn't feel natural. After a while I began using my gut instincts. It was what I called "the blood barrier", when you go from a conscious level of thinking about something, then it flips into your subconscious. With continued use, it operates in more than just your subconscious. In the mastery of anything it is taking something that you think about and turning it into something automatic.'

He continues, 'There's another level where it becomes a subconscious, embedded process in your mind, something deep within you, and that's the bit I can't teach to people. This something is a black-and-white answer; it's something within your stomach which says yes or no. But I know it's better than just mastering – mastering is teaching a kid how to drive a car at seventeen. To become a Michael Schumacher, or someone who's phenomenal at anything, it's really operating at a different level and this level uses intuition.' Greg reveals that he has a certain routine that he follows every time he trades. 'If I don't follow this routine I'm gambling,' he says. 'And, when I stop thinking and switch into my intuition, that's when the real stuff happens.'

Tap into your own intuition at work

Maria came to my intuition workshop. She told me, 'I work hard all day selling advertising space over the telephone. Then I return home to my three noisy children. I don't have one moment's peace. How can I fit practising tapping into my intuition at work?' I gave her this simple solution, which won't take time out of her hectic day. I instructed Maria that in future when the telephone rang, or if she called a client, she was to visualise the person in her mind – how old they were, what they looked like and the colour of their hair. I then told her to visualise their energy flowing down the phone line. The energy would tell her what the potential client wanted to hear from her and what they would purchase from her. Everyone has a subtle vibration that we can tap into and become aware of and work with in a positive way. Once you get the knack it will be invaluable and instant.

Some weeks later I received a very excited call from Maria, who told me, 'For the last four days I've been doing what you suggested at the workshop. I imagined my clients, what they looked like, and after a while I plucked up the courage to tell them that I thought they had dark hair or whatever. Can you believe I was right eight times out of ten?' A month later Maria called and told me she had received her sales figures. Her boss had given her a bonus because her figures had doubled. She told me, 'It's amazing they don't teach you things like this when you're training. Imagine how well the whole company would do if they learned to tap in.'

The phone game

The staff in Maria's office soon became intrigued by her testing out her psychic powers and they began a little game of their own. The company had five main products, so they wrote down the initial for each product. All their incoming calls fell into three categories – enquiries, orders and complaints. Each person had a phone on their desk and as soon as their phone rang they would first write an initial to represent which product came to mind. Then they would write 'E' for 'enquiry', 'O' for 'order' or 'C' for 'complaint'.

Maria told me, 'Apart from anything else, it's got everyone really buzzing, but the girls do seem to have an uncanny way of knowing just what the phone calls will be about.' Several people in the office turned their noses up at the 'game' and, interestingly, their orders stayed the same. However, for the girls who played the game, the ones who were tapping into their Instant Intuition, the orders went up. Now this could be because they were having so much fun that the clients reacted to them in a more positive way. But there is no escaping the fact that often these women knew just what the phone call was about and so were mentally prepared to cope with it effectively and close the deal.

Recognising your gut instinct

Using your gut instinct at work can pay dividends later. Aaron, a high-flying advertising executive, confided, 'I went for a new job and they offered it to me on the spot. It was an amazing package, yet something was stopping me from taking it. I should have signed immediately but I kept holding back. It was as if I was worrying but without knowing what about or why.' Aaron later found out the company's money was being embezzled by one of the directors. The seemingly very successful company soon went into liquidation.

Over and over again I've noticed that when clients come to see me for business reasons it's because something is niggling them. They often have no logical reason for the feeling but it exists and it won't go away. Sophie, an artist, told me, 'After our parents died their house was sold and my brother and I decided to invest our share in a property, which we would do up and let out. It seemed like the perfect investment but something kept bothering me. The annoying thing was, I had no idea what it was.'

Sophie's cards showed that her brother would be unreliable and difficult to deal with, as indicated by the appearance of the Knight of Wands reversed and the Hanged Man in the spread. Both these tarot depict someone who is not going to do any work and would soon bore of the task in question. There was a woman in the cards who also looked disapproving. Sophie, against her and my better judgement, went ahead with the project. She said, 'Soon after we started gutting the property, my brother met a new girlfriend and that was it. I was in the house alone night after night scraping old wallpaper off the walls while my brother was out wining and dining his new girlfriend. I was furious and the girlfriend turned her nose up at the property and said it was a waste of time.' She later sold the house half finished, at a small profit, just to be rid of it.

The next time you find yourself feeling agitated or hesitating, stop and listen to that inner voice. What is it telling you? If you find you keep asking people for advice about a particular project or decision, stop and wonder what is making you unsure. When you want a reading or keep reading your horoscope, what are you looking for an answer to and why? This could be your early-warning alarm bell.

Case study

Karen, a district nurse who used to work on the wards, says she had this knack of knowing when someone was going to have a cardiac arrest. She says, 'I'd find myself hovering around the bed. It was awful. I'd be waiting for it to happen. They could be sitting up talking and looking just fine, but I would know.

'I would just look at them and it was just an inner sense. Something would be saying to me, "It's going to happen." At first I used to worry that I was causing it. Sometimes the patient could be ready to be discharged and they would be telling me they were feeling fine. I would think, "No, you're not."

'Now I'm a health visitor and I'm the same with the babies. The parents will say, "He's not feeding properly," and I'll reply, "That's because he has a sore throat." The parents will look at me and I can see them thinking, "But you haven't even looked at the child." I would tell them to see their GP to check and I'm always right. I'm from a long line of doctors and nurses. As far back as our family can remember there's always been someone in medicine. Sometimes I wonder if we can trace this family skill back to the days when witches healed people.'

We've seen just a few examples I've collected over the years, but I want to tell you one more story because it happened recently and also links intuition with animals. In 2005 I visited the most wonderful place called Alladale in Scotland. It's a wilderness owned by a chap called Paul, who is a conserva-tionist. He is planting a forest and putting back plants and animals such as wolves and wild boar, which should be native to the land. I've travelled a fair amount in my time and it's easy to become blasé, but as soon as I arrived late at night during a snowstorm, I felt Alladale had a special energy of its own. Part of this energy, I'm sure, is the people who work at Alladale and the dreams they have and the energy they put into the place.

On the second day of my visit, several of us went high into the mountains on the estate to hunt for deer. I'm not big on killing animals, but they have to be culled. The ranger, Innis, was polite and informative, but I could see that his ideal day was not leading around a bunch of city dwellers. He told us to dress for a day's cold hunting. 'You could be crawling through snow for some time, so dress accordingly.' His face was a picture when the Chelsea girls showed up with Gucci written on their boots and gloves!

We searched for deer for some time. Then suddenly I said, 'Innis, they're around the other side of this peak.'

A city chap who was with us looked stunned and said, 'Can you see over there from where you are?'

I replied, 'No, but I can feel they're there.'

He laughed and looked at Innis, expecting him to smirk. Innis quietly said, 'Round this peak, you say?'

I nodded. Without a word, the ranger moved the snow vehicle and drove around the peak. There in front of us were nearly 40 deer. We startled them and they ran. I admit I was surprised that Innis took on board what I had said. As we travelled back I asked him, 'Do you sometimes just feel where the deer are?'

'Oh yes,' he replied, 'sensing where the animals are is a natural part of hunting.'

Questions, qualms and queries

As you can see, many different types of people use their intuition in all kinds of work.

Case study

Debbie, a director of a major flooring company, says, 'When something is wrong in business I have a sickening feeling in my stomach. It's like a box with a churning feeling inside and I then think, "Oh, no, not that feeling." The time I really took note of it was when it happened and the company lost a big contract. While I was waiting for the news the sick feeling was saying to me, "On alert! On alert!" Now, when I have that feeling, I ask myself, "What should I be aware of? What have I missed?" I then start to investigate everything and I keep investigating until I find the problem. I will look at the people involved, I will study their motives, I will look at figures and I will keep digging until I find the issue which could jeopardise the deal.

'I also have a warm feeling which I experience around my heart, which immediately puts me at ease concerning any business deal. This feeling always tells me when something will be fine. When I get the comfort feeling I'm so sure that things will go well that it may as well be put in writing. I know absolutely that nothing will go wrong and that I don't need to worry about the situation. These feelings don't come up every week. They may not come up for a year, but when they do I sit bolt upright and take notice.'

In the last five years since this part of my business has exploded, I've developed methods to help my business clients tap into their Instant Intuition. I could probably fill several books on the subject. One of these methods I call 'The Business Niggle', and it goes to the nub of what you need to know, although it can be used for everything from signing a contract to booking a holiday or hiring kitchen fitters. It's very useful to do before you take any big decision and sign on the dotted line.

I devised it because, during my research into this area, I spoke to many businesspeople and I noticed that when something was wrong my clients would keep thinking about it – there was a niggle. Something was holding them back for signing on the dotted line. It was as if something was missing – there was something else they needed to know about the 'deal' or situation.

Many bosses have told me, 'I wanted to come for a reading because I'm about to sign a deal and it just doesn't feel right.' This is a phrase I have heard many times from the men and women in suits, and from the artistic types who own thriving companies but look as if they've been rolling around in a field. What's more, I can relate to this feeling. I have stood with paperwork in my hand about to sign a deal but something has niggled me – something has stopped me from signing. Later, it's been a good move for a variety of reasons. Yet when I was offered a deal by Piatkus Books, my publisher, I signed the contract without even reading it. In fact the owner, Judy Piatkus, said, 'The whole deal was done in less than 24 hours. It must be a record.' At the time the proposal for *Instant Intuition* was with eight publishers, yet I had no interest whatsoever in hearing any other offers – this one felt very right.

The Business Niggle

Think back to times when you have hesitated. It may have been over buying a property or signing the contract for a new job. Perhaps it was a longed-for holiday, yet once it came to putting your name on the dotted line you hesitated.

Make sure it is a time when your niggle proved to be correct. Think of such a time and then notice what it feels like. Relive the moment and become aware of what is happening. Do you feel a tension in any area of your body? Has your thinking speeded up or slowed down? Do you have a worried feeling or is it apprehension? Do you feel you need more information?

Often the feeling is one of almost searching for further information, as if there is something you don't know yet. Identify the feeling and in future, whenever you have deals to do, paperwork to sign or simply a holiday to book, sit and relax and imagine yourself signing the deal. How do you feel? Notice whether there's a trace of this former feeling. Rethink if necessary.

Inspiration and ideas

As well as using 'The Business Niggle', the other main skill needed in commerce is ideas. No matter what field you work in, from advertising to farming, ideas oil the wheels of work. Sometimes, it can be hard to come up with a solution to a problem. What you need to do is to let your subconscious mind take over and provide the answer.

You know this can be done because there will be a time when you've walked up and down your living room or office, racking your brains, then out of the blue you get a flash of inspiration. 'That's it!' This is known as 'the eureka moment'. As you are probably aware, Archimedes discovered the principle of water displacement while taking a bath and observing how the level of the liquid rose when he put his body into the water. Suddenly, he leapt out of his bath and ran naked down the street shouting, 'Eureka!' (I have found it!). But people have been experiencing the 'eureka moment' since we began to 'think' as a species. There are many stories of great writers, teachers and inventors gaining inspiration from seemingly nowhere.

You will have experienced this yourself. You have been struggling to remember something, maybe the title of a book or who was the singer of a particular song. You may even have said, 'It's on the tip of my tongue.' In other words, it's somewhere within you but at that moment you can't find it. You go about your business, then out of the blue the answer pops into your head. Yet you weren't consciously thinking about the question. In fact you had forgotten all about it, but somewhere inside you a process was going on, a searching process, much the way a computer can be searching in the background for something while you're typing a letter or reading a web page. This process happens more often than we realise and produces answers, ideas and seemingly hidden information.

This process is well known as the 'aha factor' and it works best when we have a question that needs answering, something that perplexes us. I've devised a quick and simple exercise for you that can, as always, be applied to all areas of your life, but since we are focusing on business and fine-tuning your Instant Intuition in this area, you may want to try it out first with examples that will help you with your work.

The Aha Factor

The next time you need an answer, instead of overthinking, go for a walk and imagine handing over the query to some higher force. Don't worry about how or what is dealing with your query. The answer may come from your higher self or your subconscious mind. It may come from some higher energy. The main thing is that if you let go of the query, the answer will pop into your head when you have forgotten all about it.

Actually imagine the query floating up out of your head towards the sky and beyond. Let it go. The answer will come to you when it is ready. Simple, yes, but effective. Give it a try.

One of my clients, a lady executive, told me, 'I get some of my best ideas when I'm ironing. My director complimented me on what he called "a genius idea" recently and he asked where it came from. I said, "I've been working on it for a while." There's no way I will ever tell him it popped into my head while I was ironing my son's school uniform.'

The Litmus Test

This simple exercise will focus your mind on how and when your Instant Intuition has helped you with work.

List five incidences when you've had a gut feeling about

someone or an event at work or a decision that needs to be made or a journey that has to be taken, and each time ask yourself some questions.

◆ When you heard some work news or met someone, how did you react?

◆ Was your immediate thought, 'Well that's going to be a disaster' or 'What a terrific idea!' or 'They're great'?

◆ On one side of a piece of paper write down the date of meeting, or when you heard the news, your reaction and then the end result and date, and how long it took for your Instant Intuition to manifest into reality.

◆ You may find it interesting to note what you felt each time. Did you have any sensations, such as a revulsion, when you met the person or situation you were worrying about? A warm relaxed feeling? A feeling of dread in your stomach when you heard about a decision?

◆ Did you have any weird coincidences surrounding the person or event or decision? Was the universe trying to give you an insight? For example, you may have been thinking about relocating with your firm to York. A few days later you go to the library, pick up a magazine, open it randomly and there is a feature about this particular city and what a fantastic place it is to live. Look out for the signs. Can you remember any signs like this happening for any of your five incidences?

Future trends

At times it can be difficult to make decisions. Which job should I take? What business deal should I go for? Who should I pick for my team? Which investment fields will grow and which will slump? What will be the next big thing? If you can predict future trends in business, you will do very well in life. People tend to jump on the bandwagon when it's too late, but tapping into the *Zeitgeist* and spotting future trends is another quality that keeps the best companies ahead of the game.

A good example of a businessperson who relies on his gut instinct is the talent spotter, A&R man and pop entrepreneur Simon Cowell, *The X Factor*'s Mr Nasty. He has often referred to 'relying on my gut instinct' when choosing whether or not to work with an up-and-coming artist. He simply knows which records will sell by relying on his intuition.

> 'I never get the accountants in before I start up a business. It's done on gut feeling.'
>
> Richard Branson

Case study

Detention-centre officer Ranjit says he taps into his intuition in his job all the time and he knows when there's going to be a problem with the inmates. 'On this particular day I just knew there would be trouble,' he says. 'It was Sunday and I was on bed watch and I had a feeling on the way to work. The feeling said to me, "Keep your eyes open today." I had an image in my head of one particular person and I just knew he would cause a big fight that night.

'I arrived at work and my colleague told me, "I have a feeling things'll kick off tonight." He had sensed it too. I can usually tell by looking at someone if they'll be trouble. We deal with people from all over the world and they all have different ways of expressing nonverbal communication. At first I thought I was just reading people's body language, but I realised that something tells me before I've really looked at the person what they are like and if they will be difficult. I just know as soon as I come into contact with them. Then I study their body language and what they are saying and I can't tell you how I know but I'm always right.'

Decisions, decisions!

Caroline came to one of my workshops because she needed to make a decision. She has a hairdressing salon but wanted to expand. Her friends were all telling her to go into acrylic nails, which at the time were fashionable – every girl in town had a full set of expensive flashy nails. Caroline was unsure about this investment and something held her back.

For some clarity, she visited me and we did an exercise called 'The Three Gates', and everything became clear. Caroline clearly saw dozens of nail bars and hairdressing salons offering

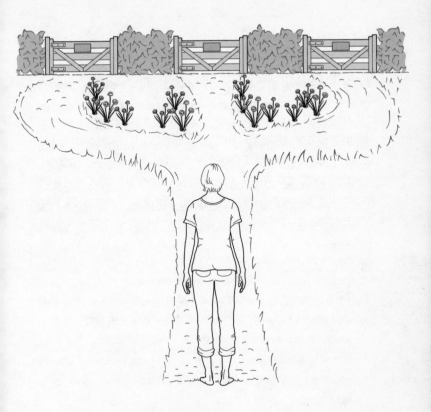

this service. She then weighed up her options and saw herself offering nonsurgical facelifts, an upmarket but nonintrusive method of firming facial muscles. Caroline's salon is booming and constantly one step ahead of the competition as she refines and updates her spa and salon treatments. 'The Three Gates' is the exercise I taught Caroline to do in order to see her options for her business. You can use this exercise when *you* have a number of options to weigh up.

....

The Three Gates

Earlier we looked at the 'Corridor' exercise in which you travelled in time. At times we have choices concerning our own destiny and this is where 'The Three Gates' is a relevant exercise. During your working life there will be times when you need to make choices. You may need to choose whether you want to work for yourself or a company. You may need to decide what to study to further your career, whether to work creatively or practically. Or you may need to chose among various jobs or decide which promotion to go for. 'The Three Gates' is an ideal exercise for making those vital decisions.

1. Take yourself to a quiet spot and relax. Allow any thoughts and issues to float to one side. Now imagine yourself in a lovely space in the countryside. It is a beautiful day with the sun shining through the trees and birds overhead, and as you look up, you see the clouds floating by driven by a light breeze.

2. Imagine yourself walking along a path and feel the grasses brush against your legs. As you smell the sweet scent of the flowers you feel at peace. Notice up in front of you there are three gates. Each gate represents a different option that you have. The gates are large and wooden, each with a blank sign. Imagine writing with a black felt-tip pen a key word to represent each option on each gate.

3. Stand back and look at the first gate and the first option. Walk up to the gate, open it and walk through. Notice any feelings you have. Can you 'see' yourself with this option?

Does this make you feel happy, wary, or can you just not imagine it happening?

4. Absorb the atmosphere and ask yourself, 'How does this make me feel?' and 'Can I see this happening?'

5. Walk back out of the gate, carefully close it, then look at Gate 2, and do the same. Remember to stop and see how it makes you feel and whether you can see anything happening. Then do the same for Gate 3.

I find that if you just cannot see or feel anything happening then it usually is not going to work out or actually happen.

Life always gives you three alternatives to any problem. I have even used 'The Three Gates' for a young woman who was deciding whether to get married. Her family were pushing her to tie the knot with one particular person but she wanted to finish her exams and wait for a few years. Her three alternatives were:

1. Get married now

2. Get married later

3. Don't get married to him at all.

I took her through all three gates and surprisingly she found that deep down she did want to marry the man, but she was angry at her family's interference and so was rejecting the option. They wed a few months later and are still very happy.

The yes/no stones

One of my favourite clients (let's call him Henry) runs one of the biggest organisations in the world and he is often seen on television. He is a Managing Director (MD) and a kind man with twinkling eyes and a natural knack for business and he uses my yes/no stones.

As I've found before in this type of situation, it was actually his PA who came to see me first for a reading and several things cropped up to do with his business that she passed on. He said very little to her but found the information intriguing enough that he booked an appointment. We had a great session and really connected, and he liked how I worked, how I used my Instant Intuition.

After this Henry would visit once a month and check out various deals and quandaries and, believe me, he had plenty! He would ask me about the competition, how certain products would fare, about future trends and about staff members. As he was running, and still does, a competitive multinational business, he needed accurate information on the spot. For years I read the cards for him monthly. Occasionally I would send him a message if something had popped into my head that I felt he needed to know urgently. But sometimes he would be overseas and with time differences and our heavy workloads, it meant we couldn't always talk. So I developed the yes/no stones so Henry could find answers quickly for himself. Perform the exercise 'The Yes/No Stones' to see how you can use them for your own guidance.

But how did I come up with the idea? I needed a tool to give to my client but instead of worrying and pushing for an answer, which I would have done years ago when Greta was alive, I 'trusted the process'. By now I knew without any doubts that it worked. I also meditated and asked for an answer – the universe does require you to put in a *small* bit of effort!

As I sat and drifted, waiting for the answer, the yin/yang symbol popped into my head. Quite why it had chosen to do so at that moment I wasn't yet sure, but I jotted it down in my spiritual diary underneath my written request to the universe: 'Please send me an instant reliable tool for Henry.'

Two days later, a client gave me a book on feng shui (the system of creating environmental balance), which explained chi, the universal life force, and how it is made up of yin and yang energy (in Chinese philosophy, yin is the negative, darker aspect, while yang is its positive opposite number). He told me, 'I have no idea why but I had a strong urge to bring you this book.' Another client, only three days afterwards, brought me a bag of crystals. She said, 'I have no idea why but I felt compelled to give you these.' I had taken time to focus and the universe had responded.

I opened the bag of crystals. Inside were five clear quartz stones, one white moonstone and one black tourmaline. I opened the book on feng shui randomly and the page said, 'Yin is dark. Yang is light. Yin is the left side of the body and Yang is the right.' I picked up the black and white stones and put one in each hand. Instinctively, I put the black one in my left hand and the white in my right, and as I did so I felt strong, balanced and at peace.

As I read more of the book I discovered that if our bodies are too yin, we need yang foods to redress the balance, and vice versa. If businesses or homes are too yang they will need yin energy.

The yin and the yang

When you visit a bachelor pad people will comment, 'This place needs a woman's touch.' In other words, it is too yang and needs some yin energy. Everything is constantly moving between yin and yang and as it flows back and forth between the two, a balance is found. When the flow is not back and forth, problems result.

The yin is feminine, right-brained, yielding, dark, cold, night, winter, receiving, passive, negative. Yang is masculine, left-brained, practical, summer, light, giving, positive, warm.

The key is to find the balance between the two and to discover when you need the yang or yin energy. Neither is right or wrong. When we say negative or positive, think in terms of a battery: it is just opposite poles, but these poles need to be in balance. Yin is thinking; yang is doing. If you are too yin you may be a bit of a dreamer and not take action. If you are too yang you will take action but perhaps not think it through properly.

Yang foods

Beef, turkey, chicken, lamb, cheese, butter, coffee, peanuts, walnuts, green peppers, onions, ginger.

Yin foods

Milk, bean sprouts, bananas, almonds, strawberries, soya beans, lemons, cucumber, cabbage, celery, fish, duck, water, tofu.

The Stones

Here is an exercise that will relieve stress while connecting you with the nature of the yin and yang stones.

1. Hold your black stone in your left hand and feel the yin energy flow up your arm and over your head. Now feel it flow down to your toes up and down the left side of your body.

2. Next, feel the white stone flow up and down your right arm, then up and down your body from the top of your head to the tips of your toes.

3. Feel the energy from the black stone flow over to your right arm and your white stone flow over to your left arm.

4. Sense the energies mingling and flowing throughout your body, and as they do so, feel balanced and connected to the universal life force. Feel strong, soft, powerful, yielding and in perfect harmony with the earth and the universe.

This exercise is particularly good when you are feeling stressed or unsettled, or you have had people drain you or make demands on you.

The Yes/No Stones

Taking the same yes/no stones, I want you to practise the previous exercise and also develop the habit of holding your stones. This will help to connect you to their energy and you will get used to feeling their subtle vibration.

1. Hold the black, negative stone in your left hand and know that this stone is your 'no' stone.

2. Hold the white positive stone in your right hand and know that this is your 'yes' stone. Feel the stone and imagine the colour and the energy flowing from the stone and into you. Feel the energy flow and notice how different each stone feels.

3. Now ask your stones a question that you already know the answer to such as:

   ◆ Am I a man?

   ◆ Am I Chinese?

   ◆ Am I wearing red?

   ◆ Does the sun come up each day?

4. Notice any feelings that occur. One stone may become hot or cold, you may have a tingling in your arm, there may be a feeling of heaviness in one of the rocks. Also, take note of when you feel something exceptionally strongly.

You can give further instructions to your stones once you are used to using them. I use the stones to tell me whether or not to take action. I focus on what I need to know, then wait to feel the answer. An energy from the yin stone tells me not to go ahead, while energy from the yang stone tells me to proceed. I feel different things at different times – maybe a slight tingle, or a heaviness or warmth in one of the stones.

I taught Henry to hold the yes/no stones and feel the energy. For me this was a big risk because I could have lost one of my best clients, but instead Henry's intuition grew to the point that people around him started to ask questions. 'How did you anticipate the competition so well?' 'How did you know which of the new products would take off and in which country?' He told them, 'I have a secret weapon.' He laughingly told me about the whispers going around the company. 'Was he using industrial espionage or tapping phones?' 'Did he have a mole working for his competitors?' He told them, 'One day I will introduce you to my secret weapon.'

And then he did. He invited me along to meet the board. So there I was, sitting at the head of a very long, expensive, polished table surrounded by men in suits. As I pulled out my tarot cards their mouths dropped open. One of the directors said, 'You've got to be kidding. You're playing a joke.' Henry said, 'Oh no, Anne is where I get my information from. Go on, ask her something.'

One of the men said, 'Okay, which car should I buy?' At that moment I had an image in my head of a brand-new Porsche. I told him, 'Not the black car – I think it's a Porsche. It's too fast for you.' The others laughed – apparently he was known for driving far too fast. The others looked interested though, if bemused, except one man who said, 'You can't expect me to take this seriously – I'm a businessman, I'm logical.' My client looked at him and said, 'And that's why I'm the MD and you're not.'

One of my major roles for Henry is to check out new staff and prospective employees. These days it's practically impossible to sack someone, no matter how bad they are at their job, and so careful selection is important. The stones quickly became popular among the board of this company to find out who they should employ. Now the directors use them in private during the interview process. But not one of these executives has told anyone in the lower ranks about the yes/no stones. They may be a little more open-minded now, but not that much.

I even have a solicitor client who keeps a stone in each pocket during difficult court cases. I am not sure what the judge, or the people he represents, would think if they knew how he was making decisions based on bits of rock. But he has told me this simple method gives him the edge.

Holistic thinker

Henry Mintzberg, of the McGill University Faculty of Management in America, conducted a large study of corporate executives. He found that the higher-level managers worked under chaotic and unpredictable conditions and constantly relied 'on hunches to deal with problems far too complex for rational analysis'. This kind of manager he termed 'the holistic thinker'. Mintzberg concluded, 'The effectiveness of an organisation does not lie in the narrow thinking of rationality. It lies in a combination of logic and powerful intuition.'

He also discovered that intuitive managers use a four-step process:

1. **preparation** – thoughts and ideas.

2. **incubation** – letting the subconscious do the work.

3. **illumination** – the answer or idea arrives in a flash.

5. **verification** – checking out how viable it is.

The undercover psychic

I want to emphasise that I do not pretend to know everything, and one area of weakness is that for some reason I am not very good at picking up on names. But I can weigh up options, so if someone is trying to work out which of several people to hire or fire, I can easily pick the best person for the job. If there is a snake in the company they can be harder to identify, which is how I started actually going into the companies and became known as 'the Undercover Psychic'.

Mr S was a director of a top software company and he knew someone was stabbing him in the back. Information was being leaked to a competitor and it was costing him dearly – they were losing business. The chairman was looking increasingly unhappy and thinking my client was not up to the job. During his reading in my office, I gave Mr S a description of the person I could feel was the sneak but it fitted several people. As he told me, 'Companies like mine are full of smart young men in suits.' I needed something more but it was just not coming through. Mr S asked me, 'Would it help if you actually came to the firm?'

I had never done this before so I wasn't sure, but hey, there's always a first time for everything, so I replied, 'I don't know but it's worth a try.'

I arrived at the company and booked in as an advertising rep. Only Mr S's trusted PA knew my real identity. Mr S called his team in and told them to run through their ideas with me for future campaigns. I sat looking knowledgeable as I listened to each one. I couldn't do anything else because I know nothing about advertising. I nodded seriously and made notes, hoping that none of them could read my mind. They all seemed like very pleasant, clever people. There was nothing that gave away a secret agenda or signs of double dealing. Whoever it was covered their tracks and bluffed very well.

Then something interesting happened. I noticed that when one particular chap – let's call him Jim – talked to Mr S his energy field drained and almost collapsed. I could see his energy field began to fade and look as if it was wilting. It became ragged at the edges. Then the colour started to drain out of his face and his body began to slump. 'It's him,' I thought to myself. Instead of trying to 'read the person' all I needed to do was watch who had the negative effect on Mr S.

If you are unsure about what I mean about seeing energy, think back to when you have seen little rainbows in a puddle. When you were a kid it looked quite magical, yet it is simply engine oil from cars on a rainy day. Just imagine the rainbow oil rippling outwards on a pond – that is a little how the aura looks around a person. Now imagine the rainbow fading into the water – this is how it looks when the person's energy drops. In my early days of watching the aura it reminded me of my gran's old oil heater. You could sit and watch waves of multicoloured heat dancing around it. (See Chapter 3 for some description of the aura.)

Later, when I spoke to Mr S, he was totally unaware that this energy drain was happening. It may come as no surprise to learn that Jim's movements were monitored and he was later sacked for gross misconduct. Following this hands-on lesson for me, I now love to watch people interacting and see how some people lift and some drain when they interact with others. It's good practice. You can add this talent to your already expanding list of skills.

'Highs and Lows'

The next time you meet a work colleague or associate for coffee, notice what happens to their energy when they talk about different people. Ask them, 'How are your family?' or maybe about various people they work with who may be shared contacts.

First, become aware of their energy field. I find that people who make us happy often create a sparkling energy. People who drain us create a dulling, almost muted, effect.

Then notice their body. Is it beginning to slump? Are the corners of their mouth beginning to turn down, or their eyes? It is amazing that they will be completely unaware of this change in their energy.

Usually people who are good for us create an upwards energy. You will see the person sit up and talk faster – their eyes will lift and their mouth will turn upwards. As they discuss people who drain them they will either become agitated or begin to look tired. I always point this out to people, especially my clients, so that they can be aware in future.

An intuitive business

Carmen Clews and Charlie Wright own and run Harlequin Marquees and Hospitality Services, a successful events company in Dubai, whose clients include Bentley, Porsche, De Beers and Burj Al Arab. In 2005 they won the International Event Professional of the Year at the annual Spotlight Awards. This award is to the events industry what the Oscars are to movies.

From Day One of their company they have used their instincts. Carmen says, 'We run our business totally on intuition. If it feels right we go with it – if it doesn't then we don't move forward. If we're not sure then we wait until we do know. No matter how much logic or facts point to something, we ignore them until our instincts show us the way.'

Carmen adds, 'When I first meet a client I get a real instinct for what will suit them. Somehow I know their tastes and what will make their event a success. What's quite interesting about "tuning in" to intuition is that, although we both ultimately come to the same conclusion, we feel it differently. For me, I usually voice all the options available to us and, as I think about or voice each one, I see what I feel. If it feels wrong I feel it niggling uncomfortably in my shoulders, and if it's the right thing then I get butterflies in my stomach. If there's no response at all, I will leave it and try not to think about it until the right answer pops into my head. This works particularly well if I have cosmically ordered the right answer to pop into my head.

'Charlie, on the other hand, feels it in his gut first, then his head makes the decision. We tend to operate very quickly. Once we have both "felt" the right decision we strongly go with it immediately without any doubts whatsoever. So, what might look like a rash decision and a risk to outsiders, to us we feel there's no losing. When it feels right, it's right and to date, it's paid off.'

Carmen says that when they get chance to switch off and go on a boat out to sea or on a trip to the mountains, where there are no distractions, that's when intuitively creative ideas pop into their heads. 'We have realisations and inspirations. Things become clear,' she explains, adding, 'Not having had any training, education or background in creating a successful business, we have had to always rely on what came intuitively. I strongly feel that this is one of our biggest reasons for our success to date.'

I wondered whether they ever disagree or have different instincts. 'Never. We always come to the same conclusions,' says Carmen. 'We pretty much bounce off each other. If I suddenly feel cautious, then Charlie will call with the same feeling.'

A good example of how they operate instinctively came when they heard a rumour that a large island in the shape of a palm tree, now called Palm Island, was about to be built along the coastline of Dubai. When plots went up for sale they put down a deposit. Charlie said, 'We had no idea what we were getting into, where to get the deposit or even a mortgage. This had never been done before in Dubai but our gut told us to go for it.' They doubled their money within a week.

Case study

Elaine is an event designer at Harlequin Marquees and Hospitality Services in Dubai (see 'A business that trusts the process'). She says, 'Working for a company which uses intuition is brilliant. It's a complete contrast to my previous existence in London's world of advertising. In my old job every decision was based on logic, and creativity was allowed only within the confines of the client's brief.

'But Charlie and Carmen have taught me to trust my intuition. At Harlequin we are constantly observing a "flow", which is reassuring, fun and powerful. This novel approach, which has become the norm for me now, reduces the levels of stress because you do your best on a physical and mental level, fulfilling your tasks with regard to the job, etc, and then you leave the rest to the universe.

'There are countless times when working on a project, something may not go exactly according to the plan, but without fail this leads to a better solution for us, the client and the business. Carmen takes this all in her stride and never doubts that everything will work out. She's amazing, and it always does in the end.'

Everyone who has met Carmen notices her attitude. Undoubtedly, part of her success is not only going with the flow (or trusting the process, as Greta called it) but also using her intuition and maintaining a positive attitude. Carmen harnesses positivity in her life and approaches any situation with positivity and 'a knowledge' that everything will work out for the best, just as Greta did.

Carmen told me, 'Even if something doesn't take you the route you expect to go, it's an approach that I am witnessing for myself as successful and there will always be a reason, which may or may not become apparent later.' I agree entirely with this statement. Chew it over and ponder it, then try to put it into practice in your business and everyday life.

I've talked a lot about the corporate world, but it wasn't just the huge corporates that consulted me. Whispers of recommendation helped to grow my business further, and these days my client list includes plumbing and building firms, music companies, restaurant owners and the self-employed as well as the general public.

Once, a couple of girls came to see me. They were pretty evasive about what they actually did for a living, but I could see they met lots of people and made a lot of money. One of them in particular had a master plan for making cash quickly, then disappearing and opening a hotel. Later their boss, Naomi, phoned me and made an appointment for the following Tuesday.

Naomi was someone you couldn't miss. She drove up in a flash Mercedes and was a larger-than-life character. A big-boned, flamboyant woman, she swept into my office and, as I later turned the cards, I said to her, 'Do you work with a lot of men? I keep getting visions of numerous males coming and going.' She roared with laughter and said, 'I should hope so. I'm the madam of a number of very successful brothels.'

I loved reading for them, partly because they were so colourful and full of interesting stories, some of which turned my ears pink. But also because I felt quite protective towards them. In a reading I could warn them about dangerous clients, police raids and unscrupulous boyfriends who were after their money. Eventually, they moved to another part of the country, which was booming, for richer pickings.

Even though I had a wide range of people coming to see me, I was surprised when a policeman called Johnny appeared at my office for a tarot reading. I was even more surprised when he told me that he often had strong gut reactions concerning cases. He said, 'I can look at someone and just know that they are guilty or hiding something. My bosses have put me on to interrogation because I get so many confessions. It's as if I'm told what to say to them to get the right information.'

Johnny said that he would know if something big was going to happen that day. In fact, he would take the feeling into consideration and 'not make arrangements in case I had to work late'. I assumed this was unusual, but time after time policemen and -women who came to see me told a similar story when I asked them about their intuitive skills. I believe they possess the same instinct as soldiers, that their sense of danger is heightened and more refined. It's an ability that the majority of the population have allowed to go dormant. If we were all in dangerous situations on a regular basis we would also become more aware.

However, not all people working in an official capacity are open-minded. Michelle, a customs officer, came to see me. I had been giving her readings over the years, but on this particular occasion she revealed, 'My boss really gives me a hard time about visiting a psychic. He believes it's all nonsense.' She told me he made comments like, 'So why can't these people tell you something useful, like who to pull out of the crowd as they walk through NOTHING TO DECLARE?'

I told Michelle that I never take the bait and try to convince people. We have to allow everyone to believe what they feel is right. But as I began my little speech, a clear image came into my mind. I told her, 'Tell your boss to look out for a man who is slim and wearing a beige suit. He has crooked teeth and a big ring on every finger. You can't miss him.' Mary went back and gave her boss the message. She rang and told me, 'He laughed in my face.'

Later that day though, they watched on a screen as a stream of people passed through customs, and a slimly built man in a beige suit walked through the NOTHING TO DECLARE gate. Michelle's boss said, 'Hey, look.' He zoomed in on the screen and became visibly pale. 'Look at his hands. He has a ring on every finger.'

Michelle piped up, 'Yes, and his teeth look a right mess.'

I never found out what the man was carrying, but he was arrested and charged. Michelle told me, 'My boss never says a word about you now. I did suggest once he should go and see you but he just walked out of the room.'

I am telling you these stories not to crow about how good I think I am but to highlight that in the business world, men and women do use their intuition. In many cases it's likely people use this sense unconsciously. But tapping in can increase the power tremendously. Why not trust your gut instinct and see what happens?

CHAPTER 8

Sweet Dreams: Waking up to Your Sleep Messages

As I approached my 50th birthday, the incredible variety of people who came for consultations kept me on my toes. In my line of work I obviously meet people from all sections of society. As well as business high-flyers, I have people from the worlds of sport, media and showbusiness on my client list, as well as unmarried mums of three. I love my work, and enjoying the way you make a living is a blessing. Part of my success is down to my attitude of trusting the universe. By the time I hit the big five O, I fully understood this concept and a strange thing began to happen to me. The more I 'let go', the fewer problems appeared in my life.

Also, after years of chain-smoking and many unsuccessful attempts to give up, I suddenly stopped. I woke up one day and thought, 'I don't want to smoke any more.' I threw my cigarettes, ashtrays and lighters away. I remembered Greta telling me, 'You'll stop smoking when you're ready to get rid of the smoke screen.' I never knew what she meant but now I had found complete inner freedom and inner peace.

As my thoughts became clearer, even more wonderful people began to appear in my life – influential thinkers whose books I had read, people I had seen on television and in newspapers and dreamed of meeting one day. A network of positivity exploded in my life and the girl who played in the backstreets in Notting Hill began to think about writing a book. I put the idea out to the universe and I knew it would happen when the time was right. I had finally realised that the universe delivers not by dropping a big cheque on our doorstep, or by sending the perfect partner by post. Instead we're given the tools we need to bring us what we want or need at that point. It is up to us to use these tools or gifts, to help us achieve our dream and not expect everything to fall into our laps.

Greta had told me to go with the flow and Vikram laughed as he told me, 'If you flow like the river you will arrive at the right bank. If you struggle you will arrive at the wrong place and you will have swallowed a lot of dirty water.' These are wise words. But I still had one psychic niggle. My dreams were becoming clearer, more frequent and more vivid. 'This has to mean something, but what and why is this happening?' I asked myself. Over the years I had tried to analyse my dreams – when I remembered them. I had bought a number of books and I had tried numerous methods but somehow dreaming that I was surfing down Slough High Street on an ironing board wearing a tutu wasn't in any of the texts. In fact, *most* things I dreamed about were not in the books.

On the odd occasion they were in the books, it didn't make much sense to me and I really wanted to understand and use the power of my dreams. I read so many stories of people gaining great insight from their night-time travels but mine seemed to be nothing more than gobbledegook.

Strange meeting

A few months after I hit fifty, I had a particularly odd dream. It was one of those dreams that stay in your mind all day. The dream hadn't been about anything that interesting, to be honest – it was short and dull – yet I couldn't get it out of my mind. I had dreamed that I had looked out of my bedroom window and below had seen my car, an old bright red Vauxhall Viva which I had bought for £180, next to Tony's flash Saab 900 turbo. By now Tony and I had split up, so it was strange that I was even dreaming about him. It had been an amicable parting. Often he was away for months, usually overseas, and we didn't have email and text – sometimes our only contact was a weekly phone call. As you can imagine, our lives took different directions and we became very different people. I hadn't dreamed about him for ages, so that was even more strange. I decided to go for a walk to clear my head and ground myself, and I fed the ducks by the river. I then went for a coffee and watched people bustling about trying to cram as much into their day as possible. It was at this moment I had a rather strange encounter.

I must have been staring into space because suddenly I heard a voice say, 'Penny for your thoughts.' I looked around to see an elderly gentlemen at the next table. He was wearing an expensive grey pinstripe suit which was frayed around the edges and he gave me a sweet smile and said, 'You were miles away.'

I found myself saying to him, 'This might sound weird but I had a dream last night and I just can't get it out of my head – yet I have no idea what it means.'

Quick as a flash he replied, 'Ah, once you can understand your dreams you open a gateway between two very different worlds.'

I wasn't alarmed that a stranger was talking to me like someone out of *The Lord of the Rings* – remember, I had opened myself up to the universe. His response made me smile because, years before, Greta had told me the same thing almost word for word, but when she was alive I could never remember my dreams, so never spent any time trying to analyse them. The coffee-shop stranger continued bringing me back to the here and now. 'Dreams can tell you some very important things. They can take you to far-off places. You can even learn to control them and make them do what you want. And, besides, some dreams are more than dreams.'

I had no idea what the comment 'some dreams are more than dreams' meant, so I gave him a quizzical look. He continued, 'I have a little method that I wish to share with you.' He took a sip of milky tea then continued, 'Most dreams are forgotten very quickly, but once in a while we have a dream that refuses to go from our minds. These dreams carry an important message. The way to unravel the message is to go back into the dream.'

This sounded interesting. 'So how do I do that?' I asked.

'Go somewhere quiet or even go back to bed,' he said, 'and allow yourself to relax, then go through the dream again and notice everything in it. If there are other people in the dream, go through it, only this time become the other person – actually *be* them. Then go back through the dream and become the objects in the dream – so if there's a chair become the chair; if there's a plane become the plane.'

The stranger sounded like a psychology professor talking to one of his first-year students. I just knew he knew what he was talking about, even though it sounded odd. I had to ask, 'If I follow this method what will it tell me?'

He paused and continued with his short tutorial. 'Each dream is different and has a specific meaning, but know that every single thing in your dream is an aspect of you – try it.' With that he stood up, smiled and bowed as if he had just conducted an orchestra, and walked out of the café. Stunned, I realised I didn't find out who he was or even his first name. I finished my coffee and popped off to the local branch of Ottakar's bookshop – I always had a quick browse before I headed home. I decided to see if there were any dream books that mentioned this technique.

As I searched through the Mind, Body, Spirit section I noticed *Great Grandfather Spirit* by Wa-Na-Nee-Chee, a Native American who travels the world spreading his message. He gave a talk in Windsor many years before and I had a vague memory of him saying something like, 'Some dreams are more than dreams – they are visions. These are the ones you cannot forget.' I flicked through his book and saw the chapter 'Dreams and Vision Journeys' which looked interesting, so I bought it and headed back to the river where I found a quiet spot.

As I flicked through, I found the relevant chapter and read about Wa-Na-Nee-Chee's thoughts on dreams. He believes dreams can reveal great knowledge and wisdom once you understand their language. They work on a psychological level which enables people to work out their problems and fears. Nightmares are our warriors. 'Strong enough to fight what you cannot face during your waking hours,' says Wa-Na-Nee-Chee. He says that if we listen to our dreams to help solve our problems, our pathway will become clear. This made sense to me and it was like a light bulb going on in my head.

When I met the stranger in the café I had mastered using intuition to tap into my own thoughts and others' feelings and emotions with EET, I had developed FLP methods that take you forward in time, I had perfected a host of other skills – and all the other techniques I've talked about in this book. Now I was clearly being given a message by the universe, with a clear sign-post from the mystery man, I needed to explore the sleeping world, the world of dreams. But my main problem was that I rarely remembered my night travels – the car story had been the first for months that had stuck in my memory.

However, that night I decided to follow the old chap's advice and go back into the dream. What did I have to lose? So I lay back on my bed and focused on my breathing and emptied my mind. If any thoughts tried to sneak in, I gently pushed them away and saw them floating off on a cloud. I went back through the dream and, because I was the only person, I followed that man's suggestion and I became my ex-partner's car. I felt powerful, fast and in control. In reality he'd had a fast flash car, so this was not that surprising. I then relived the dream and became my car. I immediately felt sluggish, lacking in power and going nowhere.

I realised how much symbolism was in the dream. The power in cars relates to their performance. But the dream was about how powerful I felt as a person at that point in my life. The dream was also symbolic of how well Tony was doing in his career and I was just plodding along. I wasn't really pushing myself. I then realised it was also a symbol of the power struggle in our relationship. Suddenly, I had a strong urge to go back into the dream and swap cars. I imagined sitting in his Saab, turning on the ignition, putting it into gear and zooming up the road. This felt good. I came out of the dream with more understanding and I felt I had reclaimed my power. This may sound simple, but I've since learned that part of the shamanic journeying technique is to reclaim lost parts of the soul that splinter off during times of trauma or upset. I had not only discovered a new psychic technique, but I felt I had retrieved some of the energy I thought I had lost for ever.

A short time after the dream, something unexpected happened. A friend who was a car dealer offered me a Saab 900 turbo. He had acquired it through a part-exchange and wanted to sell it quickly, as car dealers do, for a fantastic price. I had some spare cash and now the image in the dream had come true on another level, because I was now driving a reliable smart car rather than my old banger.

Since using this method, I've become impressed by how this stranger's technique works. I now call it *Recall Dreaming*, and I've used it to turn dreams around for myself. I think of this method as a bridge between the conscious, unconscious and the universe and I've also used Recall Dreaming to help many clients.

Recall Dreaming

1. Find yourself a comfy spot or lie down in your bed and feel yourself drift away to a special place. Take plenty of time as you allow your breathing to deepen.

2. Now relive the dream in every detail. Notice everything in it.

   ◆ How does it feel?

   ◆ What can you see?

   ◆ Are there any people in your dream?

   ◆ How do you feel about them?

3. Go through your dream and become one of the other characters and ask,

   ◆ What message do they have for me?

   ◆ What are they thinking?

   ◆ How do they relate to me?

4. Next, become each character in turn and take time to really experience what they are feeling. Are you in a building? Take in the atmosphere. Wander around and go from room to room. Remember that the building is an aspect of yourself, so become the building.

   ◆ How does it feel?

5. In your own time become everything in the dream and see what valuable insights you gain.

Case study

Lynn telephoned me from her home in Spain. She had moved to the country five years before but still kept in contact with her British friends. She told me, 'I'm perturbed by a dream about my best friend Tilly. We grew up together – she's like a sister – so I can't make any sense of this dream at all.'

In the dream, Lynn had gone to stay with Tilly. 'We were having a film-and-pizza evening indoors,' she said. 'Later that night Tilly began demanding £200 for the pizza. Next, Tilly gave me a pile of shapeless tatty clothes and began insisting that I wear them.'

I told Lynn about the technique I had learned from the stranger and she was so upset by the dream, and convinced I could help her, that a week later she flew in for a session. The dream was now reoccurring every night and Tilly was becoming more demanding in the nightmare.

Face to face, Lynn revealed that her friend Tilly had a difficult life with a violent partner and a wayward son. At times Tilly would phone Lynn distraught, and my client would invite her to stay. Often she took up her offer and enjoyed a week in the sun to recharge her batteries. They always had a wonderful time catching up and would go out on the town. Lynn introduced her to lots of people and secretly hoped that she would want to join her in Spain. So my client was astonished when she had the dream. It didn't make sense and I could see why Lynn was disturbed.

She said, 'We always go halves on everything so I have no idea why I would owe her anything. It's very upsetting.'

I put Lynn into a deep relaxation and took her back into the dream. She relived every moment, as she had seen it the first time. As with FLP, with recall dreaming she could see what was happening but this time she became her friend Tilly. Immediately Lynn said, 'Oh, she's full of resentment. When I take her out and about she feels that I'm crowing about what a lovely life I have when she's obviously struggling. I didn't mean it that way at all but I can see her point of view. I thought it would encourage her to move on, that's all.'

I asked Lynn, 'As you feel Tilly's viewpoint, what do you feel she would want to say to you?'

Lynn replied, 'We've both had problems over the years but now your life is so perfect it's not fair. My life is such a mess, which is why *you* should wear the tatty clothes. *You* should have some of the hardship I have to put up with daily. It's not fair things have turned out like this when we started in the same place.'

I then asked Lynn, 'What do you feel you would want to say back to her?'

She told me, 'I'm sorry that I've made you feel resentful. I thought I was being encouraging. But your problems are yours to sort out and face up to. It doesn't help either of us if I allow your negativity to drag me down, so I'm not wearing the tatty clothes. But I'm here for you whenever you need me.'

Lynn took a deep breath and came out of the relaxation relieved. The burden had been lifted. She called me a few months later and said, 'It's odd – on some level I feel Tilly received that message because the next time we spoke she talked more honestly about her feelings and asked my advice about getting her own life in order. She's actually doing something about her problems too, instead of moaning, which is brilliant.'

Dream on

After working with dream recall myself, and helping numerous people like Lynn, I realised the importance of dreams with regard to connecting to intuition. Sleeping is the last thing we do every day and while our bodies are sleeping and repairing, our minds are sorting out information. We wake up refreshed with our thoughts put in order and new insight into problems we've 'slept on'. The 17th-century French philosopher René Descartes, who famously said, 'I think, therefore I am', developed the idea of 'sleeping on it', which he called *dream incubation*. Descartes, who was born in 1596, was the first thinker to believe in the importance of taking control of the thinking process by planting a seed for the subconscious mind to work on during sleep.

Centuries later, many experts now agree that sleeping on a problem can produce answers that the conscious mind can't deliver. The Dutch researcher Ap Dijksterhuis, leader of psychology studies at the University of Amsterdam, found that there is an expression equivalent to 'sleeping on it' in all Western languages. In the February 2006 issue of the prestigious *Science* magazine, he remarked that the more complicated the decision, the better it was to sleep on it as opposed to examining all the facts. He said, 'It feels like it's the completely wrong way to make such an important decision. It turns out that in some circumstances it's far from suboptimal – it's the best thing you can do.'

I used to think sleep was a waste of time. I would think of all the things I could be doing instead. Now I know that without it none of us would survive. Sleep is an important process. When we don't have enough sleep we lose coordination, become grumpy, are more accident-prone and suffer from memory lapses and poor concentration. In the fifties, a popular disc jockey named Peter Tripp stayed awake for more than eight days in a glass booth in Times Square, New York, playing records. After a few days he began to hallucinate, seeing spiders and kittens, and even believed someone had dropped a hot electrode into his shoe. The stunt is believed to be so dangerous that *The Guinness Book of Records* will now not recognise it. In the laboratory, scientists have found that after five days without sleep people really do hallucinate. It's almost as if the mind *has* to dream, and even without sleep it will find a way.

> 'Sleeping has a lot of power for a lot of reasons. One is that the linear mind is shut off during sleep, so it's pure intuition.'
>
> Dr Judith Orloff, University of California

Types of dream

Below I have listed numerous types of dream – some of them I class as altered states. As you connect with your dream intuition you may want to start to keep a dream diary, just by noting down the date and a brief outline of the dream. You may be surprised at how accurate your night visions are at not only revealing your inner feelings but projecting future events.

Everyday dreams

These are the dreams that mop up all the things that have happened throughout the day. They clear our minds and organise our memories. Often an everyday dream will combine a number of the day's events. A friend of mine had a dream of cattle running through a fashion show wearing big hats. That day she had gone to a fashion show and had to drive through a small market town, where she was held up by cows crossing the road. On the journey she talked about going to the races and decided to buy herself a new hat!

Stuart Wilde, who we met in Chapter 2, has a handy technique for clearing the day's events. This is adapted from his CD *Dream Power*. As you lie in bed at the end of your day, review your day backwards. Part by part, run through all that has happened. Start with getting into bed, then go back to cleaning your teeth, all the way back to opening your eyes that morning.

Wilde says that this method clears and organises the day's events in your mind, allowing your dreams to be of a more helpful nature. He suggests you then ask a question about your future and, because you have cleared your mind, it can then work on the answer.

Years ago a girl of sixteen called Jeni popped in to see me. She said, 'I made a late appointment because this is my special dream day.' She told me that once a fortnight she stayed in bed until late morning, drifting in and out of sleep, constantly having dreams. She said, 'My special dream time really clears my head out. I feel fantastic and somehow lighter afterwards.'

Nightmares

Nightmares are purely issues and fears that we are not dealing with. Our subconscious mind is forcing us to look and be aware of what we are burying.

Telepathic dreams

We can receive messages from people or spirit guides or angels. Sometimes a message will come from someone who has passed on. This can be a great comfort to know they are still around us. Sometimes the dream gives us a warning. It can be from someone we know who is living or on the other side. My client Shirley told me, 'My husband works away on an oil rig and often he has dreams that he's talking to me. The strange thing is we often have the same dream about the same conversation. It makes us laugh because it's never anything profound, more a case of, "Have you fixed the leaking tap?"'

Recurring dreams

It can be the very same dream over and over, or dreams with a similar theme. My client Pat dreamed again and again about her kitchen, then her parents' kitchen, then her brother eating food in a kitchen. She realised the dream was to do with the family needing to nurture each other more. Recurring dreams are a nudge to alert us to an issue we need to address.

Epic dreams

These are similar to what Wa-Na-Nee-Chee called visions. They are powerful and in vivid colour. They always carry an important message which will be clear.

Daydreams

'Those who dream by day are often aware of many things which escape those who dream only by night,' said Edgar Allen Poe. Everyone daydreams. On average we all go into an altered state roughly every 90 minutes. You remember being in class and the teacher suddenly throwing the chalk at you because you were 'miles away'? Sadly, many people disregard daydreams as fantasy or time-wasting, yet they can take us into the very state we try to achieve with hypnosis or meditation. You can use daydreams to reach the inner you, get answers and improve your skills.

Many sports personalities go into a daydream state and imagine themselves playing a perfect game, which is an effective form of creative visualisation and often used in sport psychology. I think back to all the times I tried to meditate sitting cross-legged, squinting my eyes and frowning, my mind wandering – yet when that happened I was quite naturally going into this space, and I never realised it. Daydreaming is allowing your mind to go into a slightly altered state and just letting it go with the flow. It's another way to push the conscious mind to one side and get rid of logical thinking. At times this can be very useful, especially if we need new ideas or when we're stuck for an answer to something. Make no mistake, we all daydream every day. Every so often your mind will wander. It's especially common when we're driving or when someone boring is talking to us. Have you ever had that moment when someone has been talking to you and you've been miles away, then you suddenly realised they are waiting for an answer? Your conscious mind pings back into place quickly as you struggle to think of a reply.

Daydreaming plays a part in preparing ourselves for things we have to do. It is like a mental rehearsal in your mind. It is also a vital part of planning and working out how we are going to go about doing something. We make a movie in our minds. We also use it for recalling things that have happened. Daydreams can also be fantasies in which you may be scoring the winning goal at Wembley or making love to a film star. Some daydreams are about getting back at someone who has done you wrong. But I would avoid indulging in this type of mental meandering because remember, thoughts are things, and what you send out is what you get back.

How to daydream

Learn to daydream at will and you will have an extra tool in your psychic toolkit.

1. Find a comfy place to rest, maybe lie down on your bed or sink into your favourite chair. If there's something special you

need to know about, simply ask in your mind for help with the issues.

2. Put the issue completely out of your mind. It's important that you try not to think about it. Pretend you're in a special place, maybe a beautiful beach, or by a river. Notice all the sounds and colours. Look around and notice every detail. Now just relax in your special place and allow your mind to flow wherever it wishes.

3. Allow the stream of thought to flow. You may well find that an answer to your question pops into your head from nowhere or that your thinking takes you on a journey that seems totally unrelated, but stay with it. Somewhere amid the flow the answer is being worked on. It may come to you during the daydream or later in the day – but it will come.

4. Daydreaming may also give you creative ideas and innovative thinking. Practise it for a few minutes each day and your daydreaming skill will grow. By the way, if your boss asks you what you are doing, tell him you are in 'an incubation state looking for ways to make the company more money'!

....

A client who is a television producer regularly daydreams to come up with new ideas. Recently he told me, 'The pressure was on to bring in more commissions. We were working flat out but the man at the top said, "Come up with something." My secretary thinks I'm having a nap but when I'm overloaded or stressed a ten-minute daydream does the trick and puts me back on track. On this particular day, for no apparent reason, I thought of Japan. It just popped into my head. I rang a contact in Tokyo who immediately loved what I had been working on, then said he was looking for new programmes and wanted to run several we had already made and he was prepared to pay handsomely for them. My boss was very impressed.'

Premonition dreams

All ancient civilisations were aware of premonition dreams. The Greeks, Romans and Egyptians used them as a major source of information, and the ancient Babylonians made clay tablets relaying the messages received. Even today premonition dreams are still very common. People have even dreamed about winning the lottery – which you will read about in a moment.

The dream researcher and psychologist Dr Keith Hearne, the first scientist to study lucid dreaming in a laboratory, has found that there are various types of premonition dreams. One of the major classifications is what he calls 'media-announcement type'. In these, the person dreams of a television or radio news item and at some point in the future the event occurs. We tend to hear about premonition dreams mainly to do with disasters and accidents. This is probably because when something big is about to happen our primitive senses pick it up. Plus we tend to talk more about big events – we're less likely to tell everyone if we have a premonition about our friend Lucy wearing a yellow dress to a particular party.

Premonition dreams are usually useful. Sandy, a student of mine, dreamed of her husband's heart attack. She awoke feeling upset but two days later when he complained of chest pains she didn't hesitate and immediately called an ambulance, even though he was sure it was just indigestion. Her premonition dream saved his life.

Winning the lottery

You probably know someone who has had a premonition dream. Perhaps they had a vision of someone close falling ill, or dreamed the questions on an exam paper or even saw themselves wining the lottery, like Deana Sampson, whose brother visited her in a dream and gave her the winning numbers, which led to her scooping a whopping £5,439,681. Gary Ashmore picked up £1,666,667 after dreaming of becoming a millionaire while dozing at his home. He was so impressed by the power of his dream that he has since started regular consultations with a psychic.

Tammy Delph's son Jake, then five years old, also had a precognitive dream about winning the lottery. His mum explains, 'I heard him padding about on the landing and I thought he'd had a nightmare, so I asked him, "Sweetheart, what's wrong?" But rather than him saying he was scared, he told me, "Mummy, I dreamed we won lots of money, we were very rich and it was more than £50."

'I did the usual thing and said, "But we're already rich – we have each other," as I put him back to bed and settled him down. The next day Jake told my husband Malcolm about the dream. It was the first weekend of the draw in the New Year so Mal thought, "Well, you never know," and bought some extra tickets plus a Lucky Dip ticket, where the computer generates the six numbers. We won £177,356 after five numbers plus the bonus ball came up.'

Your number's up!

The best way to win the lottery is by dreaming, according to research carried out on behalf of Camelot. A survey conducted by MORI among millionaire winners discovered that an amazing 43 per cent have dreamed about their win.

Case study

Every morning, the first thing Chris, a psychic, does when he wakes up is jot down his dream. He then emails the details to the dream researcher Dr Keith Hearne. All his life Chris's dreams have come true – usually a few days later. When he was younger he had precognitive dreams two or three times a year. Now, the visions happen almost daily.

'He's provided outstanding early warning of many terrorist activities in the past, especially IRA bombings, and gave alerts just before the London bombings of 7 July [2005],' says Dr Hearne, who studied dreaming for 30 years.

'Chris receives psychic information via dreams,' explains Dr Hearne. 'The next morning he jots down anything else he can remember and then decodes the material. There are some standard symbols such as: "dogs = terrorists"; "meat = dead bodies" and "snow = imminent danger".'

For three weeks leading up to the 7 July bombings in London, Chris repeatedly dreamed of snow and dogs. On the morning of 1 July he emailed Dr Hearne and told him, 'Last night I was in a tunnel. There were two explosions, lots of soot and smoke.

There's huge great big dogs. This could be London.' Three days later he emailed Dr Hearne again: 'I've had another dream with huge dogs. I'm sure there's going to be a terrorist attack very soon.'

On 6 July the clairvoyant woke up with memories of his most disturbing dream yet. Chris, recalls, 'I saw even more mayhem. Never before had I seen so much snow – it was frozen rivers and not nice at all. There were huge Rottweilers too. That night I watched the news and prayed a terrorist attack wouldn't happen.'

But like so many times before, his precognitive dream came true. The next day he was devastated when he heard about the London bombings. 'I did let the authorities know but there was little anyone could do to prevent the attacks,' he says.

In the past Chris has made predictions, and kept records, about the Hatfield rail crash, many IRA bombs and also the Lockerbie plane crash. He adds, 'When the dreams started occurring regularly I saw my GP. I thought something was wrong with me. He told me I was insane. But I was saved by police officers and a priest who assured me that, whatever it was that was going on in my dreams, it was real. I was not mad. Now, thankfully, I work with Dr Hearne, who acts as an official, unbiased record keeper. He's got details of my visions going back 15 years.'

Alex Hall, a former detective chief inspector with the Regional Crime Squad in Luton and Dunstable, adds, 'Chris first contacted the Regional Crime Squad in 1988 with information concerning an IRA atrocity. It was treated with scepticism, as the Police have many approaches from people claiming psychic powers who are either attention seeking, misguided or whose information proves inaccurate.

'I was, however, asked by the regional coordinator to monitor Chris's dreams, which I did, sometimes on a daily basis, until I retired from the Police in 1995. As a senior police officer and experienced detective, I'd always concerned myself with hard facts and usable evidence. Because of this, Chris didn't find me an easy contact to report to, but over the years Chris has convinced me of the genuine belief he has in his powers.

'Despite the vagueness of many of his dreams, we have worked together on a number of investigations and Chris has been able to offer helpful information in relation to major crimes and terrorist activities.'

Life-saving premonitions

Mum-of-one Jackie had a terrible nightmare six years ago while on holiday in Spain. She says, 'I was in the shower when I found a lump in my right breast. I felt total terror, as if it was really happening. Then the dream whizzed forward in time to me having a mastectomy. I woke up dripping with sweat.' Unable to sleep, Jackie went over the details, but by the afternoon, she had convinced herself the nightmare was caused by something she had eaten.

But the dream resurfaced a week after she was back home. Stepping into the shower, she experienced strong *déjà vu*. 'I just had to examine myself,' she says. 'Within seconds I found a pea-sized lump in my right breast exactly as I had in my dream.' The next day, Jackie's GP told her it was probably a cyst but just to be safe referred her to a specialist. She was later diagnosed with cancer and six weeks after the dream she had a mastectomy. Last year, Jackie was given the all-clear. 'Now I think the dream was a warning and I'm so glad I acted on it. I wouldn't be here today otherwise,' she says.

But the cat nap that stunned me the most was one that Steve, the former soldier who we met in Chapter 6, had one afternoon in 2005. He dozed off in his armchair at home for just a few minutes but in that time he saw an explosion. He told me, 'I actually felt the blast and dived out of the chair. I saw a fireball and knew it was a roadside bomb and homemade, what we call an improvised explosive device. They rip cars to shreds and when these go off there are arms and legs flying.'

The dream came a few days before Steve was due to go back to Iraq to his job in security. He spent his time escorting lorries or reporters from A to B. Steve is a gifted psychic and medium and on his previous visit he gave readings to a number of chaps he was working with and told them not to leave the company they were working for because he had a gut feeling that something terrible was going to happen. Six of them had been approached by another firm, a customer who had set up his own operation to save money. Steve says, 'Even though I had a bad feeling about the whole thing, when I returned I joined the lads in the new firm. On the day we went out I told the boss, "We'll get hit today. I just know it." And that day my team got hit.'

The terrorists linked one explosive device to another so that as one went off the next one was hit as the car travelled along the road. 'As the first bomb hit us to the rear, the vehicle actually lifted,' recalls Steve. 'There was a huge dust cloud so we couldn't see anything, but I heard the second blast. The vehicle behind us had been hit.' Steve and his crew had four vehicles that were escorting five lorries in a convoy. 'It was a perfect textbook ambush,' he explains. 'Four lanes turned into one and we had to cross a bridge. Their aim was to take out the back vehicle and my vehicle to halve the protection.' As the bomb hit the second truck, a man in the back of the vehicle pointed at something, and as he did so another bomb went off under his arm and blew it clean off. Steve told me that the usual plan is to keep moving and put your foot down but instincts told him that was what the attackers wanted them to do.

'Under the bridge ahead there were about ten to 12 gunmen waiting for us. I could sense them. I knew there were more bombs ahead, out of the main killing area.' Steve's instincts kicked in. He knew not to go on but to drag the wounded man back. His men became hysterical and so he fired shots above their heads. 'I still feel guilty about firing a whole magazine over them – they looked afraid – but I knew I had to do this to get their attention and to get them to listen to me.'

He got the men to stand back-to-back so that they could protect each other from every angle, and told them not to approach the vehicle. 'I knew the enemy wanted us to go forward,' he says. 'At the moment we were hit I felt protected. Everything happened in slow motion. It was like being in [the film] *The Matrix*. One hit and I would have been gone, but I felt invincible. I felt as if I had a 20-foot angel standing over me.'

Steve forced the lads to get in an undamaged vehicle and turn back and take the injured to hospital. It was against 'orders' but he told them he would deal with the implications later. 'I felt something guiding me and shielding me,' he says. As the men drove off, their hidden attackers appeared, but it was too late – Steve and his men were speeding to safety, thanks to his dream and his intuition.

Develop Your Premonition Dreams

The best way to have premonition dreams is to focus on a particular date or event before you go to sleep. You may want to focus on next Christmas Day to see what presents you will get or whether it will snow. Focus on that day before you go to sleep. Picture it in your mind. My friend Tom focuses on horserace meetings that he will be attending. He swears that he often sees which horse will win or at least is given a clue.

Think of a time in the future when it would be useful to know what will happen. As you lie in bed at night focus on a particular date or event. It will help to visualise the daily newspaper with that date on or even a calendar on the wall with the days crossed off up to the particular day in question. So if you want to know about Christmas Day, picture your home with a calendar on the wall with the dates crossed off up to and including the 24th. Then imagine waking up that day. As you drift off to sleep your mind will focus on that point in time, and you will wake up in the morning with glimpses of what will be. Don't worry if you do not see anything on your first try. Some people need a few days to train their minds, but most will see something within a short space of time.

For most people though, as they go about their daily business, rushing here and there with their minds overloaded and surrounded by constant noise, they spare little time to listen to their own inner voice. They miss so many insights and messages because of our modern way of life, and many people have told me that they don't dream. They do – everyone dreams. You just need to know how to see, watch and listen to them.

Power naps

Some of the most logical business people are aware of what they call 'the power nap', a very brief sleep that studies have shown can refresh the mind, create ideas and solve problems – almost an instant version of sleeping on it! Thomas Edison, inventor of the light bulb, used power naps. He used to sink into his comfortable chair and place his elbow on the armrest with a handful of ball bearings. He would then drift off to sleep and, at the very moment he nodded off, his hand would relax and the ball bearings would fall clattering to the floor and wake him. This was his moment of ideas and inspirations. Winston Churchill and Margaret Thatcher both had just a few hours' sleep at night but power-napped during the day.

One night I dozed off for what must have been just a few minutes. I know it was definitely no more than five, because a programme was just finishing and when I awoke the next one hadn't started. In that short time I dreamed I was flying very high in the sky over a huge bridge. I could see cars and the lights from houses and below me an aeroplane looked as if it was about to land. I was rather like the snowman in the Raymond Briggs cartoon of that name. I awoke with a start with the thought, 'That was the Humber Bridge.' I had caught a glimpse of this structure a few years before when I had visited my friend Nicky. I certainly didn't see enough of it to recognise it but somehow I just knew this was what I had seen in my dream.

The next morning I decided to call Nicky. I'd had premonitions in the past to do with my friend, so she was quite used to odd phone calls from me. I told her my experience and she said, 'Last night at five to midnight I flew into Humberside Airport. I'd never used this airport before until yesterday.' Had I seen her trip? Had time slipped? I think perhaps I was astral-travelling, the phenomenon within which your spiritual self travels in this reality and can also go to other realms.

The following experience was even more strange for me because I do not nod off. I sleep when I go to bed, not at other times. So when I slipped away for just a few seconds in my office it seemed even more alien. I don't think I even fell asleep — it was more like suddenly going into an altered state where I found myself watching a scene as if I were looking through a hidden camera. This time, the scene I could see was my friend Carmen Clews's house in Dubai. I could see that she wasn't in, because her car wasn't outside. I could see people strolling past, the woman next door walking her dog and the passing traffic. It was dusk. Suddenly, I snapped out of the reverie and wondered why I had the images. It reminded of me when you go on the Internet and they show you 'live' footage from a city's webcam — just everyday hustle and bustle. I worked out the time difference and found that it was dusk at that moment. I emailed Carmen and told her of my vision.

She emailed me the next day saying, 'We were getting burgled at that precise time.' Dubai was voted the safest place in the world to go on holiday by *Condé Nast Traveller*, a top travel magazine, because the crime rate is almost nonexistent, so this was an incredibly unusual thing to happen. But why did I dream this at that moment? Perhaps it was because I have a connection to Carmen. Perhaps it was just more proof for me that reality isn't as straightforward as the majority of us are led to believe.

The dream I had about Carmen is very dramatic and it is a good example of a premonition vision. But by far the most usual way you will receive your psychic messages will be through symbols, like the dream I had for the top theatrical agent which you will read about shortly. Through aeons of trial and error, we know there are classical meanings for the most common dreams and I've listed these below as a quick checklist for you. If you have a particular problem, it can be helpful to write your question down on a piece of paper and fold it up. Some people like to place this under their pillow – if it works, why not?

> 'A dream which is not interpreted is like a letter which is not read.'
>
> The Talmud

Dreams and creativity

My dreams have constantly amazed me and helped me to solve dilemmas, including what to include in this book! While I'm not implying I'm Dickens, I think it's interesting to note that throughout history writers have used their dreams to create original and inspirational work.

◆ Charles Dickens commented that when he dozed he would wake up with characters in his head, which 'begged to be put down on paper'.

◆ Another writer, Robert Louis Stevenson, was inspired to write *The Strange Case of Dr Jekyll and Mr Hyde* after a terrifying nightmare. His wife was awakened by his screaming and, after she had shaken him, Stevenson angrily told her, 'Why did you wake me? I was dreaming a fine bogey tale.'

The dream was so powerful he could not rest until he had put it down on paper. It took him just three days.

◆ Musicians have inspiration dreams too. Paul McCartney composed the song 'Yesterday' after waking up one morning with the tune and the words fully formed and crystal clear in his mind.

'All my inventing, my producing, takes place in a pleasing lively dream. Dreaming is perhaps the best gift I have my Divine Maker to thank for.'

Wolfgang Amadeus Mozart

It's not just artists who receive inspiration from the divine. Albert Einstein said all his life's work came from an initial dream, which included his theory of relativity. In the dream, which ultimately changed the course of modern history, he was speeding downhill on a sledge moving so fast he was approaching the speed of light. However, you don't have to be a genius to use dreams to help you solve issues in your own life. Using this way of working is something I teach all of my students because it is so accurate, simple and instant.

Once you have mastered a few simple techniques you will have answers waiting for you most mornings, as well as inspired ideas and spiritual guidance. Dreams will also give you creative ideas that were previously way off your radar. You may wake up with an idea for a book, song or television programme. You may be inspired to design or invent something original that previously you would have had no idea of unless working with your Instant Intuition.

If I'm trying to find out some hidden information for a client, or I'm searching for the answer to a problem or dilemma, I use a method I've called 'The Dream Machine'. This technique is basically 'sleeping on it' with that little something extra. In the morning the information, or solution, is in my mind, sparkling and clear. The 'Dream Machine' exercise hands over your query to your Higher Self, which works on the answer while you sleep. This method has the benefit of bypassing your conscious mind and while you sleep the mental clutter is swept aside allowing your higher self to do its job.

'The Dream Machine' often results in out-of-the-box thinking. Many creative people get bogged down by other people's ideas or what they believe you should or shouldn't do. The creative world thrives on fresh innovative ideas and 'The Dream Machine' can provide you with a constant flow.

It's not just creativity 'The Dream Machine' can help you with. You may have a dilemma about how to handle another person – perhaps an unreasonably demanding colleague, partner or friend. One of my clients used 'The Dream Machine' to gain advice on how to deal with her mother-in-law, who would say she felt ill every time my client and her husband wanted a night out – they lived in the same house. Night after night the couple stayed in. With the help of 'The Dream Machine' my client saw her mother-in-law standing in a big field watching others picnic and having fun. The dream clearly showed that the only thing wrong with her mother-in-law was that she was lonely. They encouraged her to make a few friends, join some local societies, and suddenly her 'illness' cleared up.

The Dream Machine

1. Write down what you need to know. This can be a solution to a problem, the outcome of an event or guidance or direction. You may want inspiration, perhaps for a song, painting or story.

2. After jotting down your request, read it aloud three times before you go to sleep.

3. Place the paper under your pillow and know that your subconscious mind is going to find you the perfect answer.

Many people wake up with a song, picture, or solution that is exactly what they were looking for but couldn't connect with in their waking state.

Sometimes I have a dream, unexpectedly or intentionally, for someone else. My clients, who are often executives, people in the public eye and even MPs, take note if I tell them I've had a dream for or about them. Experience has shown that my dreams will give them vital information.

I once left a message for a top theatrical agent, saying, 'I've had a dream about the business deal you're doing.' He called me back quickly. He knew it would be important. I knew he had been negotiating with a top American network with a view to placing several of his best acts with them. We had previously consulted the cards and all looked well on the surface – yet in reality nothing was happening. Three months had passed and his contact was saying all of the right things. His contact at the network loved all of the agent's ideas, but nothing was moving forward and no deals were being signed.

I decided to use 'The Dream Machine' to find out what was happening. So before I went to sleep I focused on my client, the television network and his contact. I asked, 'What is the delay?' and I wrote it down to emphasise the question while thinking, 'Something just isn't gelling and we don't know what it is or why.' That night I had a dream that was short and simple. I dreamed that the woman the agent was dealing with suddenly had her hair hacked off. I saw her with short little tufts all over her head. The key to this method, as with all intuitive ways of working, is to take your first impressions. My immediate thought when I woke up and recalled the dream was, 'Ah, she's like Samson – she has no power.'

The biblical story of Samson's losing all his power when his hair was chopped off immediately came to me. I knew in an instant that although this contact did indeed love the ideas, she just didn't have the power to make anything happen. When I told my client a few days later he leaped up and said, 'That's it. That makes so much sense. I will contact someone higher up.' Within two weeks he had his deal.

I want to point out that I don't always dream the very night I pose the question –sometimes it takes two or three days for an answer to come through, but an answer will come. By the way, if you can't remember your dreams it could be a sign that you need B vitamins. There are several reasons why B vitamins can help us to remember our dreams. One is that a lack of this vitamin can lead to restless sleep, insomnia and stress. Also the neurotransmitter in use during REM (rapid eye movements noticeable in sleeping people) is acetylcholine, which is made from the B vitamins choline and B_5. The other Bs are needed to aid the process. Also, if you suffer from sleeping problems a dream pillow (see the box below) can help due to the healing properties of the plants.

Dream pillow

In old English folklore the grannies used to make dream pillows that contained lavender, lemon balm and roses. These natural plants can help you to have a good night's sleep and in magical traditions aid dream recall. Alternatively, dot a little pure essential lavender oil onto your pillow – or put a few drops into a warm bedtime bath.

Another method I've developed which uses the power of sleep is 'The Problem Drawer'. This technique will help you to visualise and connect on a deep level with your subconscious.

The Problem Drawer

1. As you snuggle down in bed at night feel yourself relax and almost melt into the bed. This is your haven. It's warm, soft and safe. Look around your room and know this is your space and your domain. Close your eyes and imagine that next to your bed is a chest of drawers. This chest of drawers belongs to you only. Notice how it is made of sturdy wood. Only you can open it.

2. Notice how each drawer has a label on it. Think of a problem and write a title for that problem on the label of one of the drawers. Now imagine taking a pen and paper and writing down the problem and placing it in the drawer. As you do so, feel yourself relieved of a burden. The problem is being dealt with. You have handed it over and do not need to worry about it.

3. Do the same with each problem you wish to deal with. (Some people prefer to deal with just one problem at a time.) Snuggle down and sleep soundly and know that the universe is taking care of things for you.

4. The next morning when you awake, stay in your cosy haven and slowly open a drawer in your mind. Each drawer will contain an answer. It may be something written on a piece of paper, a symbol, a person or even a message that comes directly into your mind.

It is important to stay still and cosy until you have opened each drawer. With practice you will receive answers and guidance that were almost impossible to obtain during your waking hours. The more you use your chest of drawers, the clearer the information will become.

....

Altered states

I feel lucky because I have the time and space to listen to my inner voice and I feel blessed by the people who have crossed my own path on my journey of self-realisation, my many amazing mentors. Some have come into my life for a short while, perhaps just to deliver one simple message. Others have been around for many years, perhaps even many lifetimes. They have all taught me something. At times it would be a stranger, like the man in the café who was the catalyst for my dream breakthrough, and I have learned that the key is to be aware. Once we are aware and more open, the more messages and guidance can come through in the form of Instant Intuition.

'Dreams pass into the reality of action. From the actions stems the dream again; and this interdependence produces the highest form of living.'

Anaïs Nin

I still work with Steve and Dave, the ex-soldiers we met earlier. Steve had become very involved with spiritualism and often has a timely message for me. One day as we sat drinking tea he suddenly said, 'I don't know what this means but I have to give you this message, "Not all dreams are when you are sleeping."' Steve shrugged but at that moment I had an intense moment of self-realisation, an epiphany. It suddenly clicked that I had been barking up the wrong tree during all those early years when I had tried to go into a deep trance. Instead, the occasions when I had been lost in thought, or was miles away looking out of the window of a train, or engrossed in a movie, or walking or daydreaming, letting my mind wander and ponder, I was in an altered state.

Suddenly everything became clear. Learning to tap into 'the

waking sleep' was one of my major lessons. I thought back to how Dr Helen Wambach, who we met in Chapter 5, had called her regression and progression sessions 'a waking trance', a process of simply letting your mind flow freely. I like to think that when I was told off at school for daydreaming I was actually preparing for my life's work. Or when my family said, 'She's in a world of her own', they were right – an inner world that would eventually answer everything I would ever need to know. I thought of the many ways people had tried to reach different levels of awareness, such as those who have taken mescaline and other drugs to gain spiritual knowledge. I believe that we have moved beyond this position. We don't need to take drugs to reach that level. We can do it with the power of our own minds. I believe that the human race is evolving faster than ever before and we are discovering capabilities that were previously impossible to imagine and we are also discovering our Instant Intuition.

Those who have compared our life to a dream were right … We were sleeping wake and waking sleep.'

Michel de Montaigne, 1580

Final Word

There is nothing overly dramatic about Instant Intuition — it's subtle. You won't suddenly find yourself levitating or being able to see through walls! It's simply the first thought that pops into your head when you wake up in the morning, a niggle, a tension in your tummy or perhaps an unsettling feeling around certain people. The more you begin to recognise these psychic nudges, the more you will know how to act on their information and use them to guide you in your life and importantly, the less you will feel in the dark about your relationships with others and situations.

Few of us can go and sit on top of a mountain, or at the feet of a guru or spend months on expensive courses. Today enlightenment comes when we are in a traffic jam or waiting for a train. I began my psychic quest as a child and now, in my fifties, I can look back and see the incredible difference it has made to my life.

Over the years I've read hundreds of esoteric books and I've studied dozens of techniques and the teachings of many great masters. But in truth, I learned more from Greta and Vikram than from any guru. Trial and error have given me my own techniques and many of these I've shared with you in *Instant Intuition*, my first book. My best and most accurate methods have come from thinking, 'How can I find out what I need to know?' or 'I wonder what will happen if I try this.' I am sure you will find and develop techniques of your own too, now you have a solid foundation to build on and explore.

I believe I was born no more psychic than the next person. I still fidget when I try to meditate and I am the first to admit that I don't know everything. But I promise you this – my intuition constantly steers me in the right direction, gives me answers and guides and protects me. Some of my techniques have come from my dreams, where I feel I am being given a helping hand from a higher source. Often I have tried something because quite simply I really needed an answer and knew no other way of getting it. Luckily, the answers came and continued appearing and my life has got better and better.

I've spent years trying out dozens of different methods, which I've condensed down to the absolute cream for you. I know you're busy and I know you need instant results. You don't have time to waste on the wrong partner or the wrong job. Few of us can afford to waste money on a car, house or holiday that will turn out to be wrong for us.

Throughout *Instant Intuition* I've taught you many techniques. In chapter 1 'The Album' helped you to discover who you are picking up on when you have an intuitive feeling. We also looked at stilling the monkey mind, which will bring clarity to your insights, and you learned how to use your psychic antennae, which is like having your own radar system that gives a little bleep when it needs to alert you to something significant.

In Chapter 2 we looked at opening up to allow the intuition to flow and how to close down again afterwards. You also discovered how to protect and ground yourself. Importantly, you found out how to use your intuition in your everyday life.

I introduced you to my revolutionary Etheric Energy Technique (EET) in Chapter 3, which allows you to become aware of your own energy field and use it to connect with the energy field of another person – to discover exactly how they're feeling and what they're thinking, no matter where they are in the world.

Chapter 4 looked at dowsing and its many uses, including what to eat, where to holiday and even if a couple will stay together. I even showed you how to use your pendulum to find the best place to sleep. One of the most powerful techniques I revealed in *Instant Intuition*, along with EET, is my collection of simple and safe methods for Future-Life Progression (FLP), which allow you to glimpse the future.

Do take a little quiet 'me time' to use the FLP techniques and have a peep into your own future and find out exactly where you will be and with whom, and find out what you will be doing. You can even discover who you are in your next incarnation – if you want to go that far into the future.

Chapter 6 was about using search mode and remote viewing, both of which enable you to 'see' what is happening at various locations, both near and far. Work is an important part of our lives and so I had to include the yes/no stones to enable you to boost your business intuition. Each of us has business decisions to make, whether we are a sixteen-year-old girl looking for a spare-time job in a shoe shop to get us through college or a top business person thinking of taking over a company. Each person's decision is vitally important to them, and the stones will give clear guidance.

Chapter 7 looked at using your Instant Intuition at work, and finally, we looked at dreams and the many ways you can glean information during sleep. You know now how to use 'The

Dream Machine', 'The Problem Drawer' and incubation to bring out your own inner genius and solve dilemmas. In the Appendix, there is a wealth of quizzes and exercises that will enhance your intuition dramatically.

Throughout, the book illustrates how scientists are taking a great interest in psychic phenomena and, under strict laboratory conditions, are proving that we do have an energy field, can see the future and that it is possible to discover information that is hidden by other methods. As I write this Epilogue, scientists from the University of Otago, in New Zealand, have just published a study which concludes that decisions based on gut instinct are often the best. Dr Jamin Halberstadt said in the UK press in 2006, 'There is evidence that judgements based on preference, choosing something you like, are better when made as a snap decision. When faced with choices, people make different decisions when they are asked to analyse and explain them to when they act impulsively.' For the study, volunteers had to predict the results from numerous basketball games. Half of the participants were allowed to make their choices based on statistics, while the remaining willing guinea pigs made snap decisions. Those using their gut feelings had a higher hit rate than those using logic.

While I'm not asking you to start gambling to hone your intuitive skills, I do suggest that you practise them regularly and often. You may find just doing short bursts throughout the day helpful, and you will soon find that you begin to use the methods instinctively, naturally and instantly. Undoubtedly, you will be drawn to some techniques more than others, and these will be the techniques that suit you the most and the ones that will be better for you. But do please keep practising the others too, because they will add to your range of psychic skills.

As your intuition grows, something wonderful will happen. You will find more and more coincidences appearing in your life – signposts from the universe. You may hear about a particular book three times in one day – which is a nudge that it's on the very subject you need to read up on. Or you may come across the name of someone who has a service you need or who can help you. It may be that you notice that a place or particular location keeps popping up.

A client who came on one of my workshops was thinking about buying a second property in the seaside town of Saltburn in Cleveland, but was unsure about the financial risk. Do you know what helped make up her mind (apart from the fantastic location)? Saltburn's park is called the Valley Gardens. The client spent most of her childhood in a park called the Valley Gardens 300 miles away. She spotted the subtle 'green light' from the universe and now has a great financial investment. As you recognise and take heed of the coincidences in your own life, you will connect even more to your own intuition.

Use your intuition daily as I do naturally without thinking, and watch what happens. Just a few minutes every day will do more for you than any amount of soul searching. Little by little, your skill will get stronger until you will absolutely know something without a shadow of a doubt. You will recognise a certain feeling that tells you this is good or bad, exciting, dull or dangerous. The sensation will become so powerful that you will have no doubts in your mind whatsoever. As it has for me, your Instant Intuition will become a way of life.

Over time my client base has grown bigger and bigger and for years I've had positive feedback from people I've helped face to face. My workshops have also helped many men and women bring their own intuition to the surface, who instead of spending years trying to tap into their psychic skills have done so in just one day. Imagine that! After only 24 hours they are up and running using the techniques day in and day out and regularly calling me to say, 'Guess what – I had this odd feeling about someone and . . .' or 'I use my EET to connect with my partner and . . .'

I have been running workshops for over 20 years. Time and time again I have seen people take these techniques and use them with remarkable effect. But it was when clients began contacting me with stories of their successes after I helped them from a distance that I knew it was time to go on to the next level of writing a book and pass on the techniques I have been privileged to be given.

My Instant Intuition has brought me a long way. It has changed my life by helping me with health issues. It has warned me against certain people and shown me exactly who to have in my life and who to avoid. It has brought wonderful people into all areas of my world and it has given me a wonderful career meeting people from all walks of life while taking me all over the world.

I truly hope these techniques do the same for you. Thank you for taking the time and effort to read *Instant Intuition*. There are many books on the shelves, so I am honoured that you bought mine.

Watch this space. I have a feeling this is just the beginning. I am developing and trying new methods all the time, which I will be sharing with you on my website, www.instantintuition. com. As you discover your own insights and have your own remarkable experiences please do feel free to share them on the Instant Intuition forum. I would love to hear from you.

APPENDIX

Test Your Psychic Powers

Often, people see their intuition as something vague that pops up once in a blue moon. By doing the following tests you will be able to identify your skills and hone them further. You may find that you have abilities you didn't realise you possessed. It's worth repeating these tests from time to time – you may find that some new skills appear as you develop and others become stronger.

It's a good idea to keep a log of your results and any psychic experiences you have had since starting to develop your Instant Intuition. Make sure you date each log entry so you can refer back to it.

Test 1: What is your strongest psychic sense?

Everyone has a dominant sense and by finding yours you will discover how to get the best from your intuition. You may be a good all-rounder but one sense will definitely be stronger than the others.

Read the following questions quickly and circle the most appropriate answer. At the end of the test you will discover whether you are: clairvoyant (seeing), clairsentient (feeling), clairaudient (hearing) or an empath (empathising on a deep level). You may even have a combination of these different psychic skills.

1. **When you daydream do you see clear visual images and sharp colours?**
   Yes/No/Sometimes

2. **Have you ever seen very fast-moving sparks? These usually appear as tiny pinpricks of light.**
   Yes/No/Sometimes

3. **If I say the word *elephant*, what is your response? Do you see a picture of an elephant in your mind's eye or do you see the word *elephant*? Or even both? Try this a few times with different words. Do you see an image or the letters?**
   Yes – I see an image/No – I see the word/Sometimes – I see both

4. **As you settle down to go to sleep, do random images pop into your consciousness, pictures of things that don't make sense?**
   Yes/No/Sometimes
   TOTAL: _____

5. **When you're drifting off to sleep do you ever hear voices, or the sounds of people chatting, when you are alone?**
   Yes/No/Sometimes

6. When you're frightened or feel out of your depth does a voice pop into your head and tell you, 'Don't worry, it's going to be fine' – or words along those lines?

Yes/No/Sometimes

7. Do you hear noises that you can't explain? These don't have to be voices, they could be bangs, scratches, even rustling newspaper.

Yes/No/Sometimes

8. Do you ever think your partner or friend has come back and called your name, or even just hear the door bang, only to go downstairs and find you are alone?

Yes/No/Sometimes

TOTAL: _____

9. When someone close to you is away on a trip, or even just out of the house, do you just 'know' what they are doing at a given point in the day? You may have had instances when you can remember your Instant Intuition tapping into your loved one. For example, you knew your partner was on the beach at precisely 3.30 PM – and when they rang you later this was confirmed.

Yes/No/Sometimes

10. Do you ever think about an emotional event, either personal or in the news, or sense something big is about to happen, then find it's occurred soon afterwards?
Yes/No/Sometimes

11. Do you just know what problems are going to come up in something you've planned, even before they occur?
Yes/No/Sometimes

12. Do you ever have bad feelings about a person or event that later come to fruition?
Yes/No/Sometimes
TOTAL: _____

13. Do you ever feel as if you've understood a close friend or partner or even a pet with just a quick glance? It's as if you've picked up an instant telepathic message.
Yes/No/Sometimes

14. When you are chatting with friends, do you know what they are going to say next?
Yes/No/Sometimes

15. Do you ever pick up on how strangers are feeling – happy, sad, angry, whatever?
Yes/No/Sometimes

16. **Do you ever have an urge to talk to strangers, for example on the bus, at the supermarket or in the gym?**
    Yes/No/Sometimes
    TOTAL: _____

The answers to Test 1

For every 'Yes' answer, give yourself three points, for 'No' zero and for 'Sometimes' two points. Add up your marks and note which area has the highest result. You'll have noticed that the questions are in groups of four

1 to 4: a higher mark for these four questions shows your strongest sense is CLAIRVOYANCE.

5 to 8: if you scored well in this section you are CLAIRAUDIENT.

9 to 12: a strong result here shows a gift for CLAIRSENTIENCE.

13 to 16: indicates that you are EMPATHIC.

For a detailed outline of these gifts, see Chapter 3, pages 74–6.

You may be interested to know that when two empaths meet they often form an immediate bond and find that they can almost read each other's mind. Within a short space of time they usually both pick up on people or situations around them. The information is bounced back and forth, resulting in detailed and accurate assessment. I recently introduced two empathetic friends of mine. Their conversation soon became like this: 'I wonder if that man over there is okay,' with the response, 'I was just thinking the same thing – there's something about him that's not quite right.' I listened in amusement as the other friend answered, 'Yes, I feel he's upset or worried about something. Maybe we should strike up a conversation with him.' An empath can often spot that someone is upset a mile away.

Many doctors and people in the medical profession are empaths but often suppress this talent and use logical diagnosis. They have been drawn to healing people but over time their skills can be lost among their training and what they are taught to do. A doctor who uses both skills usually ends up loved by both patients and colleagues.

Test 2: What type of psychic are you?

My specially devised quiz will instantly highlight whether you are most suited to being a healer, medium, astrologer, numerologist or tarot or palm consultant. Some of the questions may not seem relevant but they give clues to your personality and aspects of you that you may not be aware of at the moment. Simply work your way through the list and answer yes or no.

My advice is to do this test quickly without thinking too much. Take the instant answer that pops into your head – remember, you are tuned into, or are tuning into, your instant intuition!

1. When decorating, do you prefer to design the colours and layout yourself?
2. Do you prefer working to a set routine?
3. Do you like animals?
4. Are you easily distracted?

5. Do you buy clothes that are comfortable rather than fashionable?
6. Do you get bored with mundane tasks?
7. Are you an adventurous cook?
8. Do you like parties?
9. Do you feel you are different?
10. Do you get the urge to speak to someone you do not know?
11. Do you like crossword puzzles?
12. Do you daydream?
13. At school, did you prefer English to maths?
14. Do others think you are eccentric?
15. Does complicated and intricate work absorb you?
16. Do you regularly think about the past?
17. Are you the first to notice when someone is unhappy or ill?
18. Do you believe in fate?
19. Are you interested in science?
20. Do you have a good imagination?

The answers to Test 2

Make a note of the questions you said yes to – these highlight your psychic abilities. Now, look below to see how your answers match up to the different gifts (e.g. 'yes' to question 19 indicates you would be good at astrology and numerology). You may find that you score highly in more than just one category, which shows you are a good all-round psychic.

ASTROLOGY AND NUMEROLOGY
19, 15, 11, 2, 18

THE HEALING ARTS
17, 12, 5, 3, 10

MEDIUMSHIP
9, 4, 16, 20, 14

TAROT, PALMISTRY, RUNES
1, 6, 7, 8, 13

Test 3: How psychic are you?

I believe everyone is psychic to some degree and I hope this book has helped you to boost your strengths and develop your weak points. Here's your chance to find out your own ESP rating. Do the quiz now, and again in about six weeks' time, and see if your score has improved.

1. Do you dream in colour?
A. No, black and white – but I do remember some of my dreams.
B. Yes, sometimes I dream of things in colour.
C. I can barely remember last week's events, let alone my dreams.

2. What type of person are you mentally?
A. Very logical and organised.
B. Artistic and creative, a budding Picasso, actually.
C. My mind jumps from one thought to the next.

3. **If you were to meet a long-lost friend by chance, what would be your reaction?**

A. Great, I've been thinking about them over the past few days too.

B. What a coincidence! But then, it's not that strange since it's a small world.

C. Excellent! They can give me back that £10 they owe me.

4. **What type of opinions do you have when you meet someone for the first time?**

A. I don't make snap judgements. I wait until I get to know someone.

B. I instantly like or dislike people.

C. My gut instincts are usually spot-on but I've been wrong in the past.

5. **Do you believe in luck?**

A. No, you create your own good fortune.

B. Sometimes – a few strange things have happened to me.

C. Yes, whatever I need turns up.

6. **Have you ever had a bad feeling visiting a particular place or house?**

A. Occasionally, but only if I'm tired and I put it down to being tired and cranky.

B. No, I'm no Derek Acorah either – I'd be the last person to go around 'picking up vibes'.

C. Yes, and I stay away from people who make me feel drained – they're psychic vampires.

7. **What do you see when you relax and look at a clear blue sky?**

A. People's faces, animals, shapes of angels – all sorts, really.

B. The odd outline of something but mostly just meaningless shapes.

C. Clouds – big white fluffy ones.

8. **If you're feeling stressed, do you have problems with your electrical equipment at work or home?**

A. Sometimes – for example, my computer crashes for no reason and things break down.

B. Yes, I get electric shocks from things like light switches and the TV.

C. Never, and the fuses rarely blow, either.

9. **Have you ever seen a ghost?**

A. Yes, I've had several close encounters with the supernatural.

B. No, and they don't exist.

C. No, but I have a feeling of being 'watched' sometimes and put it down to my imagination.

10. **If you get lost driving, what action do you take?**

A. I never get lost, I've a strong sense of direction.

B. Look at a map or stop and ask someone the way.

C. Just follow my nose – I always get there in the end.

11. **Do you know who's on the phone before you answer it?**

A. Yes, it happens to me all the time.

B. No – but it's unplugged at home because I like peace and quiet and I'm avoiding my mother.

C. Now and again but only because I was expecting the person to call.

12. What is your opinion of ESP?

A. I'm open-minded but not totally convinced.

B. I believe in psychic abilities 100 per cent.

C. It's a complete load of rubbish. Only desperate people are interested in this type of thing.

How psychic are you?

1. (A) 2 (B) 3 (C) 1
2. (A) 1 (B) 3 (C) 2
3. (A) 3 (B) 2 (C) 1
4. (A) 1 (B) 3 (C) 2
5. (A) 1 (B) 2 (C) 3
6. (A) 2 (B) 1 (C) 3

7. (A) 3 (B) 2 (C) 1
8. (A) 2 (B) 3 (C) 1
9. (A) 3 (B) 2 (C) 1
10. (A) 2 (B) 1 (C) 3
11. (A) 3 (B) 1 (C) 2
12. (A) 2 (B) 3 (C) 1

12 points: There's not a ghost of a chance that you're remotely psychic – but that's exactly what you wanted to read, wasn't it? Lighten up and free your mind – you never know, you may enjoy it!

13 to 18 points: You show signs of psychic ability, and are open to laying a good foundation for your skills but are still letting your logical brain either block your experiences or dismiss them. If you want to hone your skills, reread the exercises in Chapters 1–3 and try them afresh before tackling the book's later techniques.

18 + points: You have definite ESP potential, but then, you knew that already. Perhaps it's time to take the next step and do a workshop. Or if you prefer to work in a group, you could join what's called a development circle, where you'll be taught how to increase your gifts. The National Federation of Spiritual Healers (NFSH) will be able to put you in contact with a local reputable psychic, who will be teaching other novices. Contact NFSH on 0845 1232777 or go to http://www.nfsh.org.uk.

How to develop your ESP – and the questions for Test 3 explained

1. People who dream in colour are usually more psychic and have a great ability to 'see' psychic images in their mind's eye.

2. Creative people are more likely to be psychic, since they're more in tune with the right side of the brain, which controls intuition, feelings and creativity. The left side of the brain is responsible for things such as planning, logic and knowledge.

3. People with a close connection share a telepathic link, even if they don't realise it, and often know subconsciously when they'll meet.

4. Trust your gut reaction. If it's not spot-on, use it more rather than block it out.

5. Optimists are more likely to have ESP abilities – including some gamblers, who may be able to influence the fall of the dice using the power of their mind.

6. Negative energy can be stored in places, mediums believe. People who are sensitive to their surroundings are psychic – even if they don't know it.

7. Letting your imagination go and seeing shapes in everyday things from the sky to brickwork to wallpaper builds up

your creative visual skills and trains the right side of the brain, the part hooked into intuition.

8. Intense emotions such as stress and anger can trigger energy transference – you may be affecting machinery unintentionally with the power of your mind.

9. If you've had a spooky encounter, you're definitely suscep-tible to clairvoyance, but just because you've don't see things, it doesn't mean you're not psychic.

10. Following your nose when travelling shows you have a natural instinct the same as natives when they 'feel' where the buffalo are, or which direction danger is coming from.

11. Telepathy often exists between close family and friends.

12. If you don't believe in anything of a psychic nature, you're unlikely to have any ESP-related experiences. But even if you did, you probably wouldn't recognise them.

The psychic museum

The world's first Psychic Museum, full of experiments to test clairvoyant powers, has just opened to the public in York, North Yorkshire. It's the brainchild of the astrologer Jonathan Cainer and the psychic celebrity Uri Geller, and is full of hands-on equipment that measures everything from a person's telepathic powers to their energy fields.

www.psychicmuseum.com or call 0800 138 9788 (UK only)

Test 4: How to spot whether your third eye is opening

As you become more aware of your own powers there will be telltale signs that your abilities are being awakened. These signs are nothing to worry about and they're all perfectly natural and part of the process of waking up spiritually. Of course, the main giveaway will be that things you just 'know' will come true. But there will also be more physical clues to look out for both physically and spiritually. You may experience one or two, or all of the following.

◆ **A tingling in the area of your third eye, which is in the middle of your forehead between your eyes**: This is a sign that your third eye (your all-seeing psychic eye) is opening.

◆ **Tension in your solar plexus**: This is your gut feeling coming into use. This can be a tingle or something much stronger. Our exercises will teach you how to define good gut feelings and warning gut feelings.

◆ **A feeling of cobwebs across your face, especially when you are trying to sleep**: This is a common sign that your spirit guides and friends are communicating with you. Take note of your dreams.

◆ **Feeling exhausted**: You are either overdoing things or you may be tapping into someone who is draining. Use the protection exercise from Chapter 1.

◆ **A tight band around your head:** You are opening psychically but need to become a little more grounded using our grounding exercise (see p. 43).

◆ **Feeling light-headed or dizzy**: Again, you need to ground yourself.

Test 5: Is your dream intuition switched on?

Read each heading and write down what you think it means. You will find the answers on the following pages. Don't peep – it will spoil the fun.

The mountain
You're halfway up a steep mountain or cliff face. You need to decide whether to carry on, even though it may be very difficult or even dangerous, or to climb back down to safety.

Water
Dreams including water can feature anything, including lakes, the sea, floods and even a swimming pool. You will be swimming easily or floating. Alternatively you may be drowning, struggling or having difficulty staying afloat – jot down what you think this means, too.

Flying
In this dream you are flying through the air. You could be zooming at a high level or close to the ground.

Falling

This can be a frightening dream. You experience plummeting from a great height perhaps from a building, cliff or bridge.

Running

You find yourself being chased by anything from the army to a monster. This dream can be terrifying or exhilarating and often you wake up with your heart pounding.

Loose teeth

Many people dream their teeth are either loose or are falling out.

The house

You find yourself wandering around a house that is either familiar or strange, roaming from room to room, or floor to floor.

Birth or babies

You're giving birth and are aware of a newly born infant that needs taking care of and you are responsible.

Nudity

Appearing naked in public without your clothes is a classic. Alternatively, you may just be wearing your underwear.

Tests and exams

Sitting at a desk, you're about to take some form of test or exam and you're panicking. You don't know the answers or you can't read the paper.

Answers to Test 5

The mountain

You have a difficult situation, or issue, in your life and you don't know whether to go forward or backwards. Keep going and you will achieve your aims.

Water

Water relates to our emotions. Deep water is thought to be dangerous. Icy or cold water depicts feelings that are being withheld or suppressed. Rough seas are difficult times ahead. Floods relate to when we feel overwhelmed by situations. A pool or pond can be calming unless it is stagnant, in which case you need to clear certain situations from your life. Lakes relate to deep emotions.

Drowning suggests you are being overwhelmed by events and are not coping. You need to take action so you're in control again – or you will 'go under'.

Water can also relate to our unconscious mind and so any dreams to do with water are from the deeper aspect of ourselves.

Flying

In some cases this can literally mean you have been astral-travelling in your sleep, but usually the dream is telling you to rise above a situation or that you're about to 'take off' with a project or situation. If you found the flight particularly easy and exhilarating, it can denote success in a matter close to your heart.

Falling

People dream that they are falling when they are feeling insecure. Look at what areas of your life are worrying you.

Running

You are facing a difficult situation in your life. Stop running and deal with it.

Loose teeth

A warning to be wary of saying something you perhaps should keep to yourself.

The house

Houses represent you and your inner self. Upper rooms represent your mental or spiritual self, lower rooms and basements your unconscious. Kitchens are to do with nurturing – either you need nurturing or you need to nurture someone close. Bedrooms are your sexuality. The hallway is when you are about to move into a different area in your life, such as changing your job. When you are wandering around a house in a dream it is a sign that you are searching for something.

Birth or babies

Something new is about to occur, a personal rebirth or spiritual awakening. It will change your life.

Nudity

Being naked or undressed in public is a sign that you are afraid of being exposed. Does someone know something about you that you do not want others to know? Are you afraid to speak up about something? It can also be a sign that you feel vulnerable or afraid.

Tests and exams

It's very common to have this dream before we actually take an exam or test. In this case it represents our fears. At other times it shows that we are worried about treading a new path or going into new areas and perhaps feeling that we don't know enough to guess the outcome. But plough on – success comes only to those who dare to take risks.

20 ways to practise using your Instant Intuition

These little exercises are perfect because they slot into your everyday life.

1. As the post arrives, build a picture in your mind. Do you see your usual postman or someone else?
2. How many envelopes do you see and what is inside them?
3. Think about future events, such as a wedding or next Christmas. In your mind, see what the weather is like. That way, at least you will know what to wear!
4. As you set off for work, which route stands out? Usually one will appear stronger or more vividly than the other options. There will be a reason for this choice – trust your gut instinct.
5. The very second you wake up in the morning, imagine your favourite newspaper's front page and 'see' the headline. Don't try to guess what it will be or think about things that have been happening recently. Simply build a picture in your mind of the newspaper and take your first thought or image. You can also try this with a different type of publication from the one you usually buy. For example, if you usually read a broadsheet, focus on a tabloid, and vice versa.

6. Have you noticed how hairdressers always ask you where you will be going on holiday? Before your next appointment, stop and imagine your hairdresser on holiday. Where do you see them? What does it look like? When you get there, instead of them asking you, you can ask them and see if you are right.

7. When being introduced to someone for the first time, imagine what their name will be as soon as you can (before you are told) and what they do for a living.

8. Sit outside and watch the clouds. Notice any shapes that may appear and focus on what the message is. I once sat in the park planning what work I needed to be concentrating on. As I thought about workshops, I noticed a giant tick-shaped cloud giving me the go-ahead. Next, I wondered whether I should visit a wilderness lodge in Scotland. The clouds took on the shape of a mountain and then a train.

9. When you are deciding which restaurant to eat in, picture several in your mind. The one that appears as a clear mental image and stands out is the right choice. You will notice that the other possible choices will look dull – or you won't even be able to visualise them.

10. If you are looking for a new or second-hand car, sit in the seat of each vehicle. How does it feel? Can you imagine yourself driving this car to work and to visit friends? Which car feels like it's yours?

11. Pick up leaflets and business cards and hold them in your hand. What impressions do you pick up about the people or business?

12. As you turn on your computer, focus and picture your inbox in your mind. How many emails do you see? Who are they from?

13. After a meal, notice how you feel. If your mind is fuzzy or you feel tired, your subconscious mind is telling you that there is something in that meal that is not right for you.

14. When the telephone rings, stop before you pick it up and 'see' who is on the other end.

15. Sit in a coffee shop and watch the counter. As people wait to be served, think about what you could imagine them drinking. Cappuccino? Latte? Decaf or espresso? Will they take sugar or a biscuit with their drink? A sprinkle of chocolate, maybe?

16. Picture in your mind the next car to come around the corner. What colour is it? If you know the difference between a Ford and a Ferrari, try to visualise the make.

17. Before you go to sleep at night, ask yourself, 'What will happen tomorrow?' Take your very first thought.

18. When meeting friends, imagine what they will be wearing.

19. As you approach the supermarket checkout, build an image in your mind of all the tills. Now imagine speeding up the image as if it were a video on fast forward. Which one moves the fastest?

20. Use the exercise called 'The Album' technique from Chapter 1. Decide which friend to see that evening by picturing the choices in your mind. Flick through each friend's image. Who gives you a warm and happy feeling? Notice your emotional and physical reactions as each image pops into your mind.

Remember to follow your hunches, listen to your Instant Intuition and it will change your life.

Bibliography

Agor, W., *Intuitive Management: Integrating Left & Right Brain Skills*, Prentice-Hall, 1984

Backster, C., *Primary Perception*: *Biocommunication with Plants, Living Foods and Human Cells*, White Rose Millennium Press, 2003

Barasch, M., *Healing Dreams: Exploring the Dreams That Can Transform Your Life*, Riverhead Books, 2000

Barratt, W., and Besterman, T., *The Divining Rod*, *An Experimental and Psychological Investigation*, Methuen & Co., 1926; and University Books, 1968

Brennan, B., *Hands of Light*, Bantam Books, 1988

Castaneda, C., *A Separate Reality*, Penguin Books, 1971

Castaneda, C., *The Teachings of Don Juan*, The University of California Press, 1968

Dean., E., D., and Mihalasky., J., *Executive ESP*, Prentice-Hall, 1974

Farrar W. V., in Williams, T., (ed), *Biographical Dictionary of Scientists*, HarperCollins, 1994

Gladwell, M., *The Power of Thinking Without Thinking*, Allen Lane (The Penguin Group), 2005

Gladwell, M., *Blink*, Penguin Books, 2006

Green, C., *Lucid Dreams*, Routledge, 1994

Harvalik, Z. V., 'A biophysical Magnetometer-Gradiometer', *Journal of the Virginia Academy of Science*, 21 (2)., 1978

Hearne, K., Dr., *Visions of the Future*, Aquarian Press, 1989

Hess, C.W., Mills, K. R., and Murray, 'N.M.F., Responses in small hand muscles from magnetic stimulation of the human brain', *Journal of Physiology*, Vol 388, Issue 1 397–419, © The Physiological Society, 1987

Holmes Atwater, F., *Captain of my Ship, Master of my Soul*, Hampton Roads Publishing Company, 2001

Kilner,. W., *The Human Aura*, Kessinger Press, 1965

Lambillion, P., *Auras and Colours*, Gateway, 2001

Linn, D., *How My Death Saved My Life*, Hay House, 2005

Lubeck, W., *Pendulum Healing Handbook*, New Age Books, 2000

Merivale, P., *Colour Talks*, Laramar, 2000

Mintzberg, H., *The Nature of Managerial Work*, Harper & Row, 1973

Mogila, I., 'Dowsing in the Soviet Union', *Psi Research*, Dowsing in the Soviet Union, March/June 1986

Monroe, R., *Journeys Out of the Body*, Bantam Doubleday Dell, 1993

Motoyama, H., Dr., The Functional Relationship Between Yoga Asanas and Acupuncture Meridians, *Healing in Our Times*, Nov. 6, 1981

Oldfield, H., *Invisible Universe*, Thorsons, 1998

Orlogg, D., Dr, *Guide to Intuitive Healing*, Times Books, 2000

Panati, C., *Supersenses*, New York Times Book Company, 1974

Radin, D., *The Conscious Universe*, HarperCollins, 1997.

Rae, A., *Quantum Physics: Illusion or Reality?*, Cambridge University Press, 1986.

Rhine, J. B., *Extra-Sensory Perception*, Brandon Book Co., 1973

Targ, R., *Limitless Mind*, New World Library, 2004

Targ, R., and Katra, J., *Miracles of Mind*, New World Library, 1998

Wa-Na-Nee-Che and Fitzpatrick, B., *Great Grandfather Spirit*, Thorsons, 2000

Wilde, S., *Dream Power* (CD), White Dove International, 1989

Wills, J., *The Food Bible*, Quadrille, 2002

Wiseman, R., *The Luck Factor*, Talk Books, 2003

Index

Index

Note: page numbers in **bold** refer to illustrations.